CELL BIOLOGY RESEARCH PROGRESS

IMMUNOGENETICS: TOLERANCE AND AUTOIMMUNITY

CELL BIOLOGY RESEARCH PROGRESS

Additional books in this series can be found on Nova's website under the Series tab.

GENETICS - RESEARCH AND ISSUES

Additional books in this series can be found on Nova's website under the Series tab.

CELL BIOLOGY RESEARCH PROGRESS

IMMUNOGENETICS: TOLERANCE AND AUTOIMMUNITY

SYLVIE LESAGE

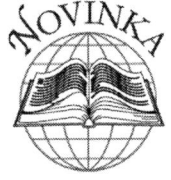

Nova Science Publishers, Inc.
New York

Copyright © 2010 by Nova Science Publishers, Inc.

All rights reserved. No part of this book may be reproduced, stored in a retrieval system or transmitted in any form or by any means: electronic, electrostatic, magnetic, tape, mechanical photocopying, recording or otherwise without the written permission of the Publisher.

For permission to use material from this book please contact us:
Telephone 631-231-7269; Fax 631-231-8175
Web Site: http://www.novapublishers.com

NOTICE TO THE READER

The Publisher has taken reasonable care in the preparation of this book, but makes no expressed or implied warranty of any kind and assumes no responsibility for any errors or omissions. No liability is assumed for incidental or consequential damages in connection with or arising out of information contained in this book. The Publisher shall not be liable for any special, consequential, or exemplary damages resulting, in whole or in part, from the readers' use of, or reliance upon, this material.

Independent verification should be sought for any data, advice or recommendations contained in this book. In addition, no responsibility is assumed by the publisher for any injury and/or damage to persons or property arising from any methods, products, instructions, ideas or otherwise contained in this publication.

This publication is designed to provide accurate and authoritative information with regard to the subject matter covered herein. It is sold with the clear understanding that the Publisher is not engaged in rendering legal or any other professional services. If legal or any other expert assistance is required, the services of a competent person should be sought. FROM A DECLARATION OF PARTICIPANTS JOINTLY ADOPTED BY A COMMITTEE OF THE AMERICAN BAR ASSOCIATION AND A COMMITTEE OF PUBLISHERS.

LIBRARY OF CONGRESS CATALOGING-IN-PUBLICATION DATA

Available upon Request
ISBN: 978-1-61761-478-1

Published by Nova Science Publishers, Inc. † *New York*

Contents

Preface		vii
Abbreviation List		ix
Chapter 1	Determining Genetic Susceptibility *Erin E. Hillhouse and Sylvie Lesage*	1
Chapter 2	T Cells *Véronique Dugas, Sylvie Lesage and Marie Vilquin*	11
Chapter 3	B Cells *Erin E. Hillhouse*	27
Chapter 4	Dendritic Cell Subsets *Sylvie Lesage, Adam-Nicolas Pelletier and Fanny Guimont-Desrochers*	37
Chapter 5	Macrophages *Véronique Dugas and Jean-François Cailhier*	47
Chapter 6	Natural Killer Cells *Geneviève Chabot-Roy, Sylvie Lesage and Fanny Guimont-Desrochers*	55
Closing Remarks		69
Index		71

PREFACE

The Human Genome Project has facilitated the identification of various genetic regions associated with disease susceptibility. This identification step is important as it yields clues into the pathways implicated in defining disease susceptibility and may uncover important therapeutic targets. Indeed, by performing genome-wide scans, one can identify many genetic loci associated with autoimmune disease susceptibility. However, the odds ratio of each locus is relatively low. Therefore, the limitation of these studies is in the biological translation of the data. This raises the question of how one verifies the true biological impact that each of these genetic variations has on human disease.

An alternative strategy for the identification of various genetic regions associated with disease susceptibility is to compare genetically resistant and susceptible individuals for biological variations. The subsequent challenge is then to demonstrate that the biological variations are causal to disease. For instance, autoimmune diseases are thought to arise as a consequence of disturbances in self-tolerance. Herein, the various mechanisms of self-tolerance, with particular emphasis on the defects potentially contributing to the onset of autoimmune diabetes, will be described. Specifically, this work will focus on the contribution of the acquired immune system and the innate immune system, including T and B cell tolerance, dendritic cells, macrophages and NK cells, as well as the potential interplay between these distinct phenotypes in defining the genetic predisposition to autoimmune diseases.

Sylvie Lesage

ABBREVIATION LIST

AICD	activation-induced cell death
Aire	Autoimmune regulator
APC	antigen presenting cells
APECED	Autoimmune Polyendocrinopathy-Candidiasis-Ectodermal Dystrophy
BAFF	B cell activating factor
BANK1	B-cell scaffold protein with ankyrin repeats 1
BCR	B cell receptor
CD	Crohn's disease
cDC	conventional DC
CFA	complete Freund's adjuvant
CLP	common lymphoid progenitors
DC	dendritic cells
EAE	experimental autoimmune encephalomyelitis
ELP	early lymphoid progenitors
eTACs	extrathymic Aire-expressing cells
GWAS	genome-wide association study
HLA	Human Leukocyte Antigen
Idd	Insulin-dependent diabetes
IDO	indoleamine 2,3-dioxygenase
IFN	interferon
iNOS	inducible nitric oxide synthase
ITAM	immunoreceptor tyrosine-based activation motifs
ITIM	immunoreceptor tyrosine-based inhibitory motifs
iTregs	induced Tregs
KIR	killer inhibitory receptor

LD	linkage disequilibrium
LOD	logarithm of the odds
MFG-E8	Milk Fat Globule-EGF factor 8
MHC	Major Histocompatibility Complex
MS	Multiple sclerosis
mTEC	medullary thymic epithelial cells
MZ	marginal zone
NK	natural killer
nTregs	natural Tregs
PAMPs	pathogen-associated molecular patterns
PD-1	programmed death-1
pDC	plasmacytoid DC
PRR	pattern recognition receptors
RA	rheumatoid arthritis
SLAM	signalling lymphocytic activation molecule
SLE	systemic lupus erythematosus
SNP	single nucleotide polymorphism
T1D	Type 1 diabetes
TCR	T cell receptor
tDC	thymic dendritic cells
TLRs	toll-like receptors
TNF	tumour necrosis factor
Tregs	regulatory T cells
TSA	tissue-specific antigens
UC	Ulcerative colitis
Yaa	Y chromosome-linked "autoimmune accelerator"

Chapter 1

DETERMINING GENETIC SUSCEPTIBILITY

Erin E. Hillhouse and Sylvie Lesage
University of Montreal, Department of Microbiology
and Immunology, Montreal, Quebec, Canada;
Maisonneuve-Rosemont Hospital Research Center, Cellular
Immunogenetics Unit, Montreal, Quebec, Canada

INTRODUCTION

Various biological processes collectively make up the immune system, which protects us from disease through the recognition and killing of foreign agents and tumor cells. However, during abnormal circumstances, the immune system mounts a hyperactive immune response against the organism's own healthy cells and tissues resulting in inflammation and tissue damage, which leads to an autoimmune disease. An autoimmune response can be specific for a particular cell type, such as pancreatic β cells in type 1 diabetes (T1D) or oligodendrocytes in multiple sclerosis (MS), but it can also target a broader range of cell types and tissues, such as nuclear antigens in systemic lupus erythematosus (SLE). Extended research throughout the years has established that both environmental and genetic factors play a role in the development of autoimmune diseases. Moreover, most autoimmune diseases are defined as complex genetic traits, since the susceptibility to disease involves a multitude of low risk factor genes.

This chapter will describe the technical advances in genetic studies, which have resulted in the identification of genetic regions associated with disease susceptibility. Specifically, we will present an overview of the execution of genetic studies as well as the advantages and disadvantages of using the genome-wide association study approach, a novel technology allowing the rapid identification of genetic loci associated with disease susceptibility.

DETERMINING GENETIC SUSCEPTIBILITY

Mouse models have been most useful in delineating the genetic factors involved in defining susceptibility to complex traits. Interestingly, both the mouse and human genomes are similarly structured with approximately 99% of mouse genes having a clear human counterpart. In fact, over 90% of the respective genomes are contained within conserved orthologous genetic segments, where genes appear in the same order on either genome. Moreover, with a century of mouse genetics [1], we now have hundreds of inbred and mutant mouse strains, which have deficiencies ranging from different stages of embryology to adulthood to a vast array of biological systems, such as the immune system, the endocrine tissues as well as the neurons. Having these various mouse strains as well as a dense genetic map at our disposal have facilitated the study of the mammalian biological system and its relevance to human conditions. A key advantage of using a live animal model is the full accessibility to affected tissue throughout progression of disease as well as prior to onset of clinical symptoms; an accomplishment which cannot readily be achieved in humans.

Because of the various benefits involved, classical genetic approaches have relied on the comparison of inbred strains to identify genetic loci associated with disease. More recently, two methods of experimentation have dominated the study of mammalian biology: reverse and forward genetics. While reverse genetics aims to define the biological function of a known gene, forward genetics describes the genes associated with a biological phenotype or function. A variety of different molecular genetic approaches can be used for either strategy. Common techniques used for reverse genetics include the use of various mouse strains to study the function of the gene in the context of a whole animal model. In particular, these include transgenic, knockout, knockdown and congenic mouse strains as well as inducible gene expression mouse models [2]. Similar strategies are applied to cell lines in order to determine the cell specific effect of eliminating or over-expressing a specific gene. Alternatively, forward genetic approaches have been extensively used in Drosophila and have been more recently applied to the mammalian system [3-

5]. Indeed, mutagen-induced point mutations which are randomly distributed throughout the genome have allowed the identification of many intracellular signaling components associated with specific phenotypes [3-5]. Therefore, both reverse and forward genetics have their independent merits, where one determines the function of a defined gene while the other uncovers the genetic description of a given phenotype. Yet, neither of these approaches efficiently identifies the genetic susceptibility of complex traits.

Nonetheless, the success of forward genetics heavily relies on the knowledge of the mouse genomic sequence and the advent of new technologies facilitating genome-wide analyses. Indeed, the availability of human genomic sequences has assisted the development of a novel technology, which is commonly referred to as a genome-wide association study (GWAS). The GWAS approach has been applied to large human cohorts and has completely revolutionized this field of research, allowing for the characterization of multiple genetic complex traits. This technique is undeniably responsible for significantly increasing the discovery rate of risk loci for many human traits and diseases, including inflammatory and autoimmune diseases [6]. Due to the prominent impact of this approach, a brief description of the strategy is provided below.

Because of the genetic heterogeneity found in humans, as opposed to inbred mice, the identification of loci that are significantly associated with a given trait of disease requires a sizeable number of patients in order to complete the study. For a GWAS, two groups are required: test subjects with the disease (cases) and similar disease-free subjects (controls). Essentially, the genome of each individual is analyzed for selected markers of genetic variation, usually for a single DNA base change, which are called single nucleotide polymorphisms (SNPs). Each SNP is linked to a known allele in the examined population and, thus, they are used as markers to define the allelic genotype of each individual. Various quantifiable phenotypes can then be correlated with the SNP results. The frequency of a given genotype is compared between cases and controls and, depending on the observed frequency of these variations in the subjects with disease, the variations may or may not be found to be "associated" with the disease. The associated genetic variations are then considered as indicators of disease susceptibility regions [7]. These regions can vary both in size, depending on the extent of the linkage disequilibrium, and in gene content [8], where the number of genes within the region can range from several to none. Moreover, a SNP located outside a coding sequence might be correlated to the causal variant located within a coding sequence, which can lead to a functional or structural modification of the protein (protein quality). It can also be associated with a regulatory variant, therefore modifying the gene expression (protein quantity). In all cases, *functional studies are needed to characterize the actual effect of the variant.*

In order to determine the significance of the genetic variation to susceptibility, a GWAS utilizes a classical logarithm of odds (LOD) score linkage analysis, where the probability of linkage between disease and marker loci is compared to the probability of no linkage. This odds ratio is then taken to determine the LOD ratio. Currently, genetic association p-values smaller than 5×10^{-8} are the accepted measure of significant association to disease [9]. Nevertheless, many factors contribute to a given susceptibility locus, making the validation of significance quite difficult and new statistical validation approaches are constantly being revised to increase the sensitivity of the GWAS [10].

In complex genetic traits, most loci will confer low risk to disease. However, in some instances, a single locus is highly associated with, and significantly contributes to, disease predisposition. In such cases, it becomes very difficult to identify other loci conferring a relatively low risk. The Human Leukocyte Antigen (HLA) in humans, or the Major Histocompatibility Complex (MHC) in mice, is a perfect example of a locus strongly associated with autoimmune disease predisposition. Although the exact association between the HLA and autoimmunity remains unclear, a common view suggests that a breakdown occurs in the immunological tolerance to self-antigens through aberrant class I and class II presentation of self or foreign peptides to autoreactive lymphocytes [11-14]. The HLA locus is one of the most extensively studied regions in the human genome because of the contribution of multiple variants at this locus towards multiple diseases. Indeed, the HLA has been associated with susceptibility to MS, T1D, SLE, ulcerative colitis (UC), Crohn's disease (CD), as well as rheumatoid arthritis (RA) [15] and has the greatest and/or most consistent genetic risk associated with these diseases in comparison to other loci linked to disease susceptibility [6]. For example, *HLA* (located on human chromosome 6) has the most significant linkage to T1D with a LOD score of 213.2 and accounts for approximately 50% of the inheritable susceptibility [12]. After the HLA, the next suggestive evidence of linkage to T1D is located near *CTLA4* and *INS* (insulin gene) with a LOD score of 3.28 and 3.16, respectively [15]. Thus, it is clear that the remaining susceptibility genes have much lower overall contributions to diabetes risk compared to the collective contribution of HLA genes. Nevertheless, *variation within the HLA locus does not explain autoimmune disease development for all subjects*, therefore, it remains important to identify and understand how susceptibility genes with lower LOD scores influence disease development. We must bear in mind that the ultimate aim of these investigations is to provide a sufficient understanding of the pathways contributing to autoimmune disease to facilitate the design of new specific therapeutic approaches related to the genotype of the patient.

Genetic association studies are limited in part by the occurrence of linkage disequilibrium (LD), where combinations of alleles at two or more loci, not necessarily found on the same chromosome, occur more or less frequently in a population than would be expected. Thus, LD measures the non-random associations between polymorphisms at different loci. As a result, if one identifies a variant that is associated with disease, it will be *difficult to determine whether the variant is causal of disease or whether its association simply reflects LD with the true causal variant*. Indeed, HLA haplotypes demonstrate strong LD. Hence, the causal HLA variants have remained vague for the great majority of diseases [12].

Regardless of advances in genetics and the increasing availability of novel genetic tools, we have yet to identify the causal gene or genes for >75% of the newly identified susceptibility loci [6]. Indeed, at least 17 genetic regions associate with lupus predisposition and each of these genetic intervals potentially represent causal genetic variants that largely remain to be discovered [16]. Moreover, of the 421 genes within the HLA, only 40% are known to be expressed, while less than one third of these genes have a defined biological function [12]. Clearly, *identifying a susceptibility region does not readily define the causal gene or mechanism*. Extensive studies are needed in order to first determine which genetic variants actually contribute to disease susceptibility followed by how these variants affect biological function and increase susceptibility to disease [17]. This task will require very strong collaborations between human geneticists and experimental biologists if we are to understand how these sequence variants influence disease pathogenesis.

Prior to the development of the GWAS, a major limitation of human genetic studies was that the technology relied on testing a small number of variants across the genome, with each study using a different set of variants and/or typing methodology. This problem has resulted in a literature base that can be complex and at times conflicting. In order to differentiate the effects of tightly linked loci, a dense map of variation is needed in *large cohorts of ethnically diverse populations*, so that rare, distinguishing recombination events can be identified [12]. Particularly, a large number of DNA markers (> 100 000 SNPs) from clinically well-defined patients and matched controls need to be genotyped. Using larger cohorts for all studies including replication studies facilitates the identification of most of the genetic variation in the human genome [6]. It should be noted that large inbred families could unexpectedly highlight the major effect of a susceptibility gene, which in a heterogeneous sample of small families displays only a minor overall effect [18].

Another limitation, which also applies to the current GWAS technology, is the *inability to replicate genetic associations in some or all subsequent studies*. This could be due to sampling variation (different samples of families from a same population containing different frequencies of susceptibility genes), population genetic variation (ethnic groups), population environmental factors leading to different levels of penetrance of interacting susceptibility genotypes, combinations of the above, or no true linkage (false positive) [18]. Indeed, a common limitation of the GWAS approach is the high potential for false-positives given the massive number of statistical tests performed. Consequently, there is a greater requirement for reproduction of results and a higher threshold of statistical significance [19].

The analysis of a GWAS must take into account that weak linkage associations could be attributed to 2 key possibilities:

1. The susceptibility gene occurs in only a small proportion of patients, or
2. The susceptibility gene produces only a slight increase in risk, suggesting the possibility that the gene acts concurrently with other genes to cause disease.

Therefore, in a given individual, the combination of these minor genes could have a stronger effect on disease development and susceptibility. Nevertheless, *weak linkage association to a particular region means that the gene itself will be difficult to locate, difficult to confirm* in independent studies and *difficult to isolate* by genetic procedures.

Finally, identification of genetic variants and molecular pathways associated with disease susceptibility through linkage analysis studies in mice compared to data obtained in humans shows that an interesting parallel can be made, at least for autoimmune diabetes, where common genes and pathways contribute to disease predisposition [20]. There are also significant advantages to using mouse models rather than humans. Mouse genetic studies take advantage of established inbred strains which simplify the genetic approach and reduce the cost. As opposed to humans, where thousands of individuals need to be genotyped to identify significant linkages, a few hundred mice are sufficient to identify multiple genetic loci associated with disease. For this approach, highly significant differences must be observed for a given phenotype upon comparison between two independent inbred strains. These strains are then interbred for two generations (F2), where these F2 generation offspring exhibit random recombination events between the two parental strains. Subsequently, the linkage analysis of the phenotype and genotype allows for the rapid identification of genetic loci, as well as interacting loci, involved in determining the phenotype. Thus, the combination of the human GWAS approach and mouse genetics may rapidly help identify key pathways regulating immune tolerance and preventing autoimmune disease progression.

CONCLUSION

The introduction of the GWAS approach has had an extraordinary impact on our knowledge of the genetics of many autoimmune diseases, bringing to light many unexpected candidate genes and biological pathways [6]. The GWAS facilitates the discovery of susceptibility genes for a given disease, where clinicians may then use these susceptibility genes to assess the likelihood of an individual in developing the disease. More importantly, identification of causal genes will increase the understanding of the disease process, which will ultimately lead to the creation of preventative therapies. However, many susceptibility loci remain to be discovered and may necessitate the generation of new tools in order to access the more infrequent variants [21]. Identification of the variants causal to disease will also require extensive investigations. Furthermore, designing methods for prevention will require that we also understand the mechanisms through which genetic susceptibility occurs and how these interact with non-genetic factors. Therefore, although genetic studies are part of the answer to developing new therapies, determining the absolute susceptibility to disease will depend on establishing the contribution of both genetic and non-genetic factors.

The following chapters will discuss the contribution of variations in immune tolerance to autoimmune disease susceptibility and the implication of genetic studies in understanding biological pathways associated with autoimmune diseases.

REFERENCES

[1] Paigen, K., One hundred years of mouse genetics: an intellectual history. I. The classical period (1902-1980). *Genetics.* 2003. 163: 1-7.

[2] Paigen, K., One hundred years of mouse genetics: an intellectual history. II. The molecular revolution (1981-2002). *Genetics.* 2003. 163: 1227-1235.

[3] Hoyne, G. F. and Goodnow, C. C., The use of genomewide ENU mutagenesis screens to unravel complex mammalian traits: identifying genes that regulate organ-specific and systemic autoimmunity. *Immunol. Rev.* 2006. 210: 27-39.

[4] Kile, B. T. and Hilton, D. J., The art and design of genetic screens: mouse. *Nat. Rev. Genet.* 2005. 6: 557-567.

[5] St Johnston, D., The art and design of genetic screens: Drosophila melanogaster. *Nat. Rev. Genet.* 2002. 3: 176-188.

[6] Lettre, G. and Rioux, J. D., Autoimmune diseases: insights from genome-wide association studies. *Hum. Mol. Genet.* 2008. 17: R116-121.

[7] Pearson, T. A. and Manolio, T. A., How to interpret a genome-wide association study. *JAMA.* 2008. 299: 1335-1344.

[8] Barrett, J. C., Hansoul, S., Nicolae, D. L., Cho, J. H., Duerr, R. H., Rioux, J. D., Brant, S. R., Silverberg, M. S., Taylor, K. D., Barmada, M. M., Bitton, A., Dassopoulos, T., Datta, L. W., Green, T., Griffiths, A. M., Kistner, E. O., Murtha, M. T., Regueiro, M. D., Rotter, J. I., Schumm, L. P., Steinhart, A. H., Targan, S. R., Xavier, R. J., Libioulle, C., Sandor, C., Lathrop, M., Belaiche, J., Dewit, O., Gut, I., Heath, S., Laukens, D., Mni, M., Rutgeerts, P., Van Gossum, A., Zelenika, D., Franchimont, D., Hugot, J. P., de Vos, M., Vermeire, S., Louis, E., Cardon, L. R., Anderson, C. A., Drummond, H., Nimmo, E., Ahmad, T., Prescott, N. J., Onnie, C. M., Fisher, S. A., Marchini, J., Ghori, J., Bumpstead, S., Gwilliam, R., Tremelling, M., Deloukas, P., Mansfield, J., Jewell, D., Satsangi, J., Mathew, C. G., Parkes, M., Georges, M. and Daly, M. J., Genome-wide association defines more than 30 distinct susceptibility loci for Crohn's disease. *Nat. Genet.* 2008. 40: 955-962.

[9] Risch, N. and Merikangas, K., The future of genetic studies of complex human diseases. *Science.* 1996. 273: 1516-1517.

[10] Jacobs, K. B., Yeager, M., Wacholder, S., Craig, D., Kraft, P., Hunter, D. J., Paschal, J., Manolio, T. A., Tucker, M., Hoover, R. N., Thomas, G. D., Chanock, S. J. and Chatterjee, N., A new statistic and its power to

infer membership in a genome-wide association study using genotype frequencies. *Nat. Genet.* 2009.
[11] Muller-Hilke, B., HLA class II and autoimmunity: epitope selection vs differential expression. *Acta Histochem.* 2009. 111: 379-381.
[12] Fernando, M. M., Stevens, C. R., Walsh, E. C., De Jager, P. L., Goyette, P., Plenge, R. M., Vyse, T. J. and Rioux, J. D., Defining the role of the MHC in autoimmunity: a review and pooled analysis. *PLoS Genet.* 2008. 4: e1000024.
[13] Harbo, H. F., Lie, B. A., Sawcer, S., Celius, E. G., Dai, K. Z., Oturai, A., Hillert, J., Lorentzen, A. R., Laaksonen, M., Myhr, K. M., Ryder, L. P., Fredrikson, S., Nyland, H., Sorensen, P. S., Sandberg-Wollheim, M., Andersen, O., Svejgaard, A., Edland, A., Mellgren, S. I., Compston, A., Vartdal, F. and Spurkland, A., Genes in the HLA class I region may contribute to the HLA class II-associated genetic susceptibility to multiple sclerosis. *Tissue Antigens.* 2004. 63: 237-247.
[14] Horton, R., Wilming, L., Rand, V., Lovering, R. C., Bruford, E. A., Khodiyar, V. K., Lush, M. J., Povey, S., Talbot, C. C., Jr., Wright, M. W., Wain, H. M., Trowsdale, J., Ziegler, A. and Beck, S., Gene map of the extended human MHC. *Nat. Rev. Genet.* 2004. 5: 889-899.
[15] Concannon, P., Chen, W. M., Julier, C., Morahan, G., Akolkar, B., Erlich, H. A., Hilner, J. E., Nerup, J., Nierras, C., Pociot, F., Todd, J. A. and Rich, S. S., Genome-wide scan for linkage to type 1 diabetes in 2,496 multiplex families from the Type 1 Diabetes Genetics Consortium. *Diabetes.* 2009. 58: 1018-1022.
[16] Harley, J. B., Kelly, J. A. and Kaufman, K. M., Unraveling the genetics of systemic lupus erythematosus. *Springer Semin. Immunopathol.* 2006. 28: 119-130.
[17] Rioux, J. D., Goyette, P., Vyse, T. J., Hammarstrom, L., Fernando, M. M., Green, T., De Jager, P. L., Foisy, S., Wang, J., de Bakker, P. I., Leslie, S., McVean, G., Padyukov, L., Alfredsson, L., Annese, V., Hafler, D. A., Pan-Hammarstrom, Q., Matell, R., Sawcer, S. J., Compston, A. D., Cree, B. A., Mirel, D. B., Daly, M. J., Behrens, T. W., Klareskog, L., Gregersen, P. K., Oksenberg, J. R. and Hauser, S. L., Mapping of multiple susceptibility variants within the MHC region for 7 immune-mediated diseases. *Proc. Natl. Acad. Sci. U. S. A.* 2009. 106: 18680-18685.
[18] Field, L. L., Genetic linkage and association studies of Type I diabetes: challenges and rewards. *Diabetologia.* 2002. 45: 21-35.

[19] Hunter, D. J. and Kraft, P., Drinking from the fire hose--statistical issues in genomewide association studies. *N. Engl. J. Med.* 2007. 357: 436-439.
[20] Maier, L. M. and Wicker, L. S., Genetic susceptibility to type 1 diabetes. *Curr. Opin. Immunol.* 2005. 17: 601-608.
[21] Manolio, T. A., Collins, F. S., Cox, N. J., Goldstein, D. B., Hindorff, L. A., Hunter, D. J., McCarthy, M. I., Ramos, E. M., Cardon, L. R., Chakravarti, A., Cho, J. H., Guttmacher, A. E., Kong, A., Kruglyak, L., Mardis, E., Rotimi, C. N., Slatkin, M., Valle, D., Whittemore, A. S., Boehnke, M., Clark, A. G., Eichler, E. E., Gibson, G., Haines, J. L., Mackay, T. F., McCarroll, S. A. and Visscher, P. M., Finding the missing heritability of complex diseases. *Nature.* 2009. 461: 747-753.

Chapter 2

T CELLS

Véronique Dugas[1], Sylvie Lesage[1] and Marie Vilquin[2]

[1] University of Montreal, Department of Microbiology and Immunology, Montreal, Quebec, Canada; Maisonneuve-Rosemont Hospital Research Center, Cellular Immunogenetics Unit, Montreal, Quebec, Canada.
[2] Maisonneuve-Rosemont Hospital Research Center, Cellular Immunogenetics Unit, Montreal, Quebec, Canada; Lille University of Sciences and Technologies, Villeneuve d'Ascq, France.

INTRODUCTION

T cells are necessary and sufficient for the progression of various autoimmune pathologies, such as T1D, RA and thyroiditis. For instance, transfer of T cells from a diabetic mouse to an otherwise healthy mouse is sufficient to induce autoimmune diabetes progression [1]. Also, in individuals affected by SLE, T cells are known to be hyperactive and resistant to apoptosis [2]. Moreover, patients suffering from RA show elevated amounts of the inflammatory cytokine IL-17, a cytokine produced by a subset of CD4 T cells [3]. Clearly, T lymphocytes are implicated in the susceptibility of these diseases as well as other autoimmune pathologies. The defects in T cell function that lead to autoimmune pathologies can result from various immune check points involved in imposing T cell tolerance to self-tissues. Some critical events in the control of T cell tolerance will be discussed below.

Moreover, we will describe how defects in T cell tolerance induction may contribute to autoimmune disease susceptibility and progression.

OVERVIEW OF T CELL DIFFERENTIATION AND FUNCTION

The thymus is a primary lymphoid organ wherein proceeds the early education of immature T cells, hereafter referred to as thymocytes. Indeed, thymocytes which recognize self-peptides with low affinity in the context of MHC class I or II molecules will differentiate into naïve T cells expressing CD8 or CD4 co-receptor, respectively. These T lymphocytes will then exit the thymus, migrate to the periphery and travel through secondary lymphoid organs in search of a pathogen. Defects in the ability of T cells to recognize pathogens and mount an efficient response lead to an impaired capacity to fight infections, which can result in deleterious consequences for the host. Consequently, the T cell responses must be intricately tuned to allow adequate recognition of pathogenic antigens, all the while precluding T cell activation upon binding to self-antigens. Consequently, both central and peripheral tolerance mechanisms are responsible for establishing this balance.

CENTRAL TOLERANCE

The role of the thymus is to generate functional T cells, while eliminating autoreactive T cells. This is achieved by way of positive and negative thymic selection processes, which collectively are commonly referred to as central tolerance. During positive selection, thymocytes with a low affinity for self-MHC peptide complexes are allowed to mature. This ensures that thymocytes which emigrate from the thymus will sufficiently recognize both self-peptide/MHC complexes, which will promote T cell survival, and pathogenic-peptide/MHC complexes presented at the surface of a professional antigen-presenting cell (APC), namely dendritic cells (DC), macrophages and B cells, which will induce an efficient immune response. On the other hand, T cell discrimination between self and non-self proteins is critical in the prevention of autoimmune reactions. Negative selection is the process that entails the elimination of thymocytes exhibiting a strong affinity or avidity for self-peptides before they escape from the thymus. Indeed, thymic DC (tDC) and medullary thymic epithelial cells (mTEC) constitutively process and present self-peptides to thymocytes. If the strength of the interaction between the T cell receptor (TCR) on the thymocyte and the peptide/MHC complex on the APC exceeds a certain threshold, the T cell will be subject to apoptosis, a tightly regulated cell death process that does not lead to inflammation. Therefore, negative selection should allow for the efficient elimination of most autoreactive T cells. Nevertheless, defects in the negative selection process will enhance susceptibility to autoimmune diseases.

In this regard, a defect in the induction of the Bcl-2 family member Bim, a pro-apoptotic mediator, correlates with impaired negative selection [4]. As suggested, $Bim^{-/-}$ animals show an increase in susceptibility to autoimmune diseases and develop severe kidney autoimmune disease (24). Moreover, Bim expression is dysregulated in autoimmune diabetes-prone NOD mice [5], a commonly used murine model that is also susceptible to other autoimmune deficiencies, such as thyroiditis and SLE [6, 7]. Moreover, abnormally low and high thresholds for positive and negative thymocyte selections, respectively, are also responsible for an increased proportion of autoreactive T cells in the NOD mouse and possibly in other mouse strains, as well [8-10].

Negative selection is also dependent on the efficiency of antigen presentation by tDC and mTECs. tDCs present ubiquitously expressed self-antigens to immature thymocytes resulting in the apoptosis of thymocytes which have a high affinity to self-antigens. Consequently, this limits the export of autoreactive T cells from the thymus into the periphery. However, not all antigens are expressed by DCs circulating in the thymus. Some tissue-specific antigens (TSA) remain sequestered within organs such as the skin, eyes, brain, pancreas, etc. It has recently been shown that mTECs specialize in the presentation of TSA to thymocytes, a mechanism regulated by Autoimmune regulator (Aire) [11]. Aire expression is mainly restricted to mTECs [12]. Therefore, defects in Aire should lead to an increase in autoimmune susceptibility to specific organs. Indeed, Aire-deficient mice develop autoimmune responses to a limited set of antigens, where the antigenic specificity is conferred by the genetic background of the mouse strain [11, 13]. More importantly, mutations in *AIRE* are responsible for causing the autosomal recessive Autoimmune Polyendocrinopathy-Candidiasis-Ectodermal Dystrophy (APECED) pathology, where patients develop massive lymphocytic infiltrations and produce multiple autoantibodies to various tissues [14-16]. Finally, Aire-deficient mice have facilitated the identification of the biological role of this protein in the induction of negative selection and tolerance to tissue-specific self-antigens [11, 17-19]. In summary, negative selection generally induces apoptosis of thymocytes that are specific for ubiquitously or ectopically expressed self-antigens. As a result, reported defects in negative selection processes have been associated with a direct increase in susceptibility to autoimmune disease progression.

PERIPHERAL TOLERANCE

Although thymic selection processes promote the maturation of T cells that are not self-reactive, a sizeable proportion of autoreactive T cells can be found in periphery. In an attempt to control autoimmune responses in the periphery, some T cells with a relatively high affinity for self-peptide/MHC complexes are spared from negative selection and undergo a distinct differentiation program which leads to immune regulation [20]. The most studied regulatory T cell population is defined as "natural" (ie: originating from the thymus) lymphocytes which express both the CD4 co-receptor and the activation marker CD25 (nTregs). In humans, as in mice, the up-regulation of the transcription factor FOXP3 is a requisite step for the differentiation and function of nTregs [21]. However, FOXP3 expression is not limited to nTregs as is also expressed by CD4 T cells which acquire their regulatory phenotype and function in the periphery, giving rise to the term "inducible" Tregs (iTregs). Indeed, in the presence of IL-2 and TGF-β and in the absence of inflammatory cytokines, naïve CD4 T cells up-regulate the expression of FOXP3 and become potent regulators [22]. Importantly, when Tregs encounter an APC presenting a peptide for which they are specific, they become activated and abrogate the proliferation of surrounding T cells via IL-2 deprivation, cell-to-cell contact and secretion of immunoregulatory cytokines, such as IL-10 [23]. Clearly, Tregs play a prominent role in peripheral tolerance mechanisms [24].

As Tregs are central to the maintenance of peripheral tolerance, it is not surprising to find that genetic defects in *FOXP3*, which precludes the appropriate generation and function of Tregs, are associated with autoimmune diseases in both humans and mice. In humans, individuals bearing mutations in the *FOXP3* gene develop a multi-organ autoimmune disease that is usually lethal before the age of 2 [25]. Similarly, the Scurfy mouse model, which carries a mutation in *Foxp3,* also presents a severe autoimmune phenotype comparable to the disease observed in humans [26]. Together, these data demonstrate that a defect in the regulation of Tregs is sufficient to confer an increased risk of developing an autoimmune disease. Despite the lack of a clear association between Treg number and the prevalence of any given autoimmune disease, several different groups have highlighted functional defects in Tregs from patients suffering from relapsing-remitting MS [21]. Moreover, many pathways associated with type 1 diabetes predisposition might affect Treg function, such as the CTLA-4 and the IL-2/CD25 pathways. In particular, the insulin-dependent diabetes 3 *(Idd3)* locus, which defines a susceptibility region for autoimmune diabetes in NOD mice, encompasses the *Il2* gene, where genetic variants of this gene have been identified [27, 28]. Although it is tempting to suggest that the biological contribution of *Il2* genetic variants alters Treg function and, thus, increases autoimmune susceptibility, the mechanism of action of the *Il2* variants has not been fully determined and is subject to debate [27-32]. Finally, even though CD4+CD25+ FOXP3+ Tregs are the most extensively studied, other subtypes of immunoregulatory T cells have also been identified for their role in tolerance maintenance, such as CD8$\alpha\alpha$ intraepithelial lymphocytes [33] and double negative T lymphocytes [34, 35]. However, their role in the prevention of autoimmune disease progression remains to be fully established.

As discussed above, mechanisms involved in the presentation of TSA are present in the thymus. Indeed, AIRE has proven to be a requisite for an efficient selection of non-autoreactive thymocytes. However, it has recently been proposed that AIRE could also be expressed in the periphery in order to further delete self-specific T cells. For instance, extrathymic Aire-expressing cells (eTACs) reside mainly in T-cell zones located in secondary lymphoid organs [36]. These stromal cells are positive for MHC class II expression and are, thus, presumably capable of antigen presentation [36, 37]. Even though it has been demonstrated that eTACs can directly interact with and delete autoreactive T cells, their precise role in autoimmune disease prevention remains to be established.

Another key mechanism which limits aberrant autoreactive T cell responses in the periphery is tolerance induction as defined by the "two signal model". This model illustrates the intrinsic activation requirement of naïve T cells to receive both a TCR signal (recognition of a peptide-MHC complex) as well as co-stimulation signals. More specifically, after emigrating from the thymus, naïve T lymphocytes circulate within lymphoid organs aiming to encounter an APC presenting an antigen for which they exhibit sufficient affinity. However, the interaction between the TCR and a peptide-MHC complex alone is insufficient to induce the full T cell activation necessary to provoke an immune response. Consequently, APCs up-regulate co-stimulatory molecules, such as CD80 and CD86, only in the presence of inflammation [38]. Naïve T cells, which constitutively express the counter-ligand, CD28, can, thus, be fully activated to induce an immune response. In absence of this co-stimulatory signal, the T cell will either become non-responsive or will become subject to apoptosis, two mechanisms of peripheral tolerance induction that are respectively referred to as anergy and activation-induced cell death (AICD). As a result, in the absence of inflammation, a potentially autoreactive T cell will either become unresponsive or will be removed from the circulation. Interestingly, deletion of co-stimulatory molecules, such as CD80 and CD86 or CD28 in NOD mice accelerates the onset and severity of autoimmune diabetes [39, 40], further highlighting the importance of tight regulation of co-stimulation for the prevention of autoimmune disease. The loss of CD80 and CD86 co-stimulatory proteins also leads to a dramatic decrease in Treg numbers in the thymus and periphery [41], which may explain part of the mechanism by which these molecules contribute to the maintenance of immune tolerance. Moreover, it should be noted that activated T cells up-regulate the expression of CTLA-4, an inhibitor of T cell activation which competes with CD28 for binding to CD80 and CD86 [42] and is directly involved in anergy induction as well as the control of Treg function [43, 44]. The expression of CTLA-4 is crucial in order to avoid lymphoproliferative disorders, as it leads to cell cycle arrest, inhibition of CD25 and CD69 up-regulation, decreased IL-2 production as well as an increased threshold for subsequent activation (56). Indeed, CTLA-4 deficiency leads to massive lymphoproliferation and multi-organ tissue infiltration leading to death within 3 to 4 weeks of age [45, 46]. This fulminant immune response to multiple tissues underlines the critical role of CTLA-4 in the induction of immune tolerance. The contribution of CTLA-4 genetic variants to autoimmune susceptibility has been confirmed in both mice and humans [47, 48]. Specifically, in NOD mice, the *Idd5.1* autoimmune diabetes susceptibility locus includes *Ctla-4* as a candidate gene. Furthermore, through recent GWAS, genetic variants of *CTLA-4* have been associated with susceptibility to numerous autoimmune diseases, including SLE, RA, Grave's and celiac diseases [49]. The biological implications for different CTLA-4 genetic variants are under current investigation [50-53].

Finally, other defects in co-stimulation pathways have been associated with autoimmunity. Indeed, PD-1 (programmed death 1) also acts as a negative regulator expressed on the surface of activated T and B cells. PD-1 is thought to be responsible for the maintenance of long term tolerance following activation, mainly by limiting T cell function [54]. Deficiencies in PD-1 are known to induce spontaneous autoimmunity in different mouse strains, notably autoimmune cardiomyopathy in BALB/c mice [55] and a lupus-like disease in

C57BL/6 mice, an otherwise auto-immune resistant strain [56]. Moreover, polymorphisms in PD-1 have been associated with various autoimmune pathologies in numerous human cohorts, pinpointing its role in tolerance induction [54].

Peripheral tolerance is also maintained by immune-regulation of the Th1/Th2/Th17 pathways. Indeed, in 1986, Mosmann showed that CD4 T cells can be separated into two distinct populations according to their cytokine production profile, namely Th1 and Th2 [57]. Th1 cells produce IL-2 and IFN-γ pro-inflammatory cytokines and promote cytotoxic and inflammatory responses, while Th2 cells secrete IL-4 and IL-10, both of which are associated with immune deviation and tolerance induction. Another pro-inflammatory subset of CD4 T cells has recently been identified and is designated Th17 for its prominent potential at producing the IL-17 cytokine, a chemotactic cytokine facilitating the recruitment of neutrophils [58]. Other than IL-17, Th17 cells also produce a vast array of pro-inflammatory cytokines, including IL-1, IL-6, IL-8, IL-22 and TNFα, which are known to recruit and activate monocytes, macrophages, neutrophils and other innate immune cells. In particular, Th17 cells have been associated with MS and RA pathologies, while Th1 contribute to T1D and MS [59-62]. Evidence that Th17 contribute to autoimmune progression has been recently revealed by various genetic deletions in molecules contributing to Th17 differentiation, such as IL-12, IL-23 and IL-25 [63, 64].

Alterations in the balance of immune-regulation in favor of Th1 or Th17 immune responses may promote autoimmunity. IL-12 and IL-21 are cytokines which respectively promote Th1 and Th17 differentiation [65-67]. Genetic variants of both of these cytokines are included within autoimmune diabetes susceptibility regions, where *Il12* is located within *Idd4* and *Il21* is included within the *Idd3* interval [68, 69]. Interestingly, the IL-12p40 gene product can pair with IL-12p35 to form the Th1 promoting IL-12 cytokine or with IL-23p19 to create the Th17 promoting IL-23 cytokine [70]. Therefore, understanding the biological role of IL12p40 genetic variants may generate interesting therapeutic targets playing a central role in both Th1 and Th17 phenotypes. In contrast, IL-21 specifically impacts Th17, not Th1, differentiation. IL-21 is also implicated in chronic infections and the generation of memory T cells [71-73], which may contribute to autoimmune progression. In autoimmune prone NOD mice, pancreatic levels of IL-21 increase during diabetes development whereas the genetic ablation of the IL-21 pathway prevents autoimmune diabetes progression [69, 74]. Together, these results suggest that an intricate balance of the immune regulation of Th subsets is at play in defining the susceptibility to autoimmune diseases.

CONCLUSION

T cells, which develop in the thymus, must recognize self-peptide/MHC proteins with sufficient affinity in order to promote their maturation and survival. Yet, they must not recognize self-peptide/MHC complexes with ample affinity to induce an immune response. This dichotomy between self/non-self recognition has been a central theme in trying to understand the role of the immune response. Other than central tolerance, which is mostly mediated by negative selection, potentially autoreactive T cells are also subject to peripheral tolerance mechanisms, such as inhibition by Tregs, anergy, AICD and immune-regulation of the various Th pathways. Both co-stimulatory molecules and cytokines are key players in the regulation of the majority of the pathways involved in peripheral tolerance induction. Here, we have highlighted evidence demonstrating that alterations in any of these pathways which facilitate T cell activation are sufficient to increase the susceptibility to autoimmune disease progression. However, it should be noted that autoimmune diseases are multi-factorial. Essentially, although genetic ablation leads to severe phenotypes, the role of subtle genetic variants encoded within the genome only slightly increases the risk of developing autoimmunity. The following chapters will describe how other cellular subsets contribute to autoimmune disease progression.

REFERENCES

[1] Haskins, K., Pathogenic T-cell clones in autoimmune diabetes: more lessons from the NOD mouse. *Adv. Immunol.* 2005. 87: 123-162.
[2] La Cava, A., Lupus and T cells. *Lupus.* 2009. 18: 196-201.
[3] Chabaud, M., Durand, J. M., Buchs, N., Fossiez, F., Page, G., Frappart, L. and Miossec, P., Human interleukin-17: A T cell-derived proinflammatory cytokine produced by the rheumatoid synovium. *Arthritis Rheum.* 1999. 42: 963-970.
[4] Bouillet, P., Purton, J. F., Godfrey, D. I., Zhang, L. C., Coultas, L., Puthalakath, H., Pellegrini, M., Cory, S., Adams, J. M. and Strasser, A.,

BH3-only Bcl-2 family member Bim is required for apoptosis of autoreactive thymocytes. *Nature.* 2002. 415: 922-926.

[5] Liston, A., Lesage, S., Gray, D. H., O'Reilly, L. A., Strasser, A., Fahrer, A. M., Boyd, R. L., Wilson, J., Baxter, A. G., Gallo, E. M., Crabtree, G. R., Peng, K., Wilson, S. R. and Goodnow, C. C., Generalized resistance to thymic deletion in the NOD mouse; a polygenic trait characterized by defective induction of Bim. *Immunity.* 2004. 21: 817-830.

[6] Many, M. C., Maniratunga, S. and Denef, J. F., The non-obese diabetic (NOD) mouse: an animal model for autoimmune thyroiditis. *Exp. Clin. Endocrinol. Diabetes.* 1996. 104 Suppl 3: 17-20.

[7] Silveira, P. A. and Baxter, A. G., The NOD mouse as a model of SLE. *Autoimmunity.* 2001. 34: 53-64.

[8] Kwon, H., Jun, H. S., Yang, Y., Mora, C., Mariathasan, S., Ohashi, P. S., Flavell, R. A. and Yoon, J. W., Development of autoreactive diabetogenic T cells in the thymus of NOD mice. *J. Autoimmun.* 2005. 24: 11-23.

[9] Kishimoto, H. and Sprent, J., A defect in central tolerance in NOD mice. *Nat. Immunol.* 2001. 2: 1025-1031.

[10] Lesage, S., Hartley, S. B., Akkaraju, S., Wilson, J., Townsend, M. and Goodnow, C. C., Failure to censor forbidden clones of CD4 T cells in autoimmune diabetes. *J. Exp. Med.* 2002. 196: 1175-1188.

[11] Anderson, M. S., Venanzi, E. S., Klein, L., Chen, Z., Berzins, S. P., Turley, S. J., von Boehmer, H., Bronson, R., Dierich, A., Benoist, C. and Mathis, D., Projection of an immunological self shadow within the thymus by the aire protein. *Science.* 2002. 298: 1395-1401.

[12] Hubert, F. X., Kinkel, S. A., Webster, K. E., Cannon, P., Crewther, P. E., Proeitto, A. I., Wu, L., Heath, W. R. and Scott, H. S., A specific anti-Aire antibody reveals aire expression is restricted to medullary thymic epithelial cells and not expressed in periphery. *J. Immunol.* 2008. 180: 3824-3832.

[13] Jiang, W., Anderson, M. S., Bronson, R., Mathis, D. and Benoist, C., Modifier loci condition autoimmunity provoked by Aire deficiency. *J. Exp. Med.* 2005. 202: 805-815.

[14] Peterson, P., Org, T. and Rebane, A., Transcriptional regulation by AIRE: molecular mechanisms of central tolerance. *Nat. Rev. Immunol.* 2008. 8: 948-957.

[15] An autoimmune disease, APECED, caused by mutations in a novel gene featuring two PHD-type zinc-finger domains. *Nat. Genet.* 1997. 17: 399-403.

[16] Mathis, D. and Benoist, C., Aire. *Annu. Rev. Immunol.* 2009. 27: 287-312.
[17] Anderson, M. S., Venanzi, E. S., Chen, Z., Berzins, S. P., Benoist, C. and Mathis, D., The cellular mechanism of Aire control of T cell tolerance. *Immunity.* 2005. 23: 227-239.
[18] Liston, A., Lesage, S., Wilson, J., Peltonen, L. and Goodnow, C. C., Aire regulates negative selection of organ-specific T cells. *Nat. Immunol.* 2003. 4: 350-354.
[19] Liston, A., Gray, D. H., Lesage, S., Fletcher, A. L., Wilson, J., Webster, K. E., Scott, H. S., Boyd, R. L., Peltonen, L. and Goodnow, C. C., Gene dosage--limiting role of Aire in thymic expression, clonal deletion, and organ-specific autoimmunity. *J. Exp. Med.* 2004. 200: 1015-1026.
[20] Andre, S., Tough, D. F., Lacroix-Desmazes, S., Kaveri, S. V. and Bayry, J., Surveillance of antigen-presenting cells by CD4+ CD25+ regulatory T cells in autoimmunity: immunopathogenesis and therapeutic implications. *Am. J. Pathol.* 2009. 174: 1575-1587.
[21] Brusko, T. M., Putnam, A. L. and Bluestone, J. A., Human regulatory T cells: role in autoimmune disease and therapeutic opportunities. *Immunol. Rev.* 2008. 223: 371-390.
[22] Chen, W., Jin, W., Hardegen, N., Lei, K. J., Li, L., Marinos, N., McGrady, G. and Wahl, S. M., Conversion of peripheral CD4+CD25- naive T cells to CD4+CD25+ regulatory T cells by TGF-beta induction of transcription factor Foxp3. *J. Exp. Med.* 2003. 198: 1875-1886.
[23] Vignali, D. A., Collison, L. W. and Workman, C. J., How regulatory T cells work. *Nat. Rev. Immunol.* 2008.
[24] Sakaguchi, S., Yamaguchi, T., Nomura, T. and Ono, M., Regulatory T cells and immune tolerance. *Cell.* 2008. 133: 775-787.
[25] Bussone, G. and Mouthon, L., Autoimmune manifestations in primary immune deficiencies. *Autoimmun. Rev.* 2009. 8: 332-336.
[26] Bennett, C. L., Christie, J., Ramsdell, F., Brunkow, M. E., Ferguson, P. J., Whitesell, L., Kelly, T. E., Saulsbury, F. T., Chance, P. F. and Ochs, H. D., The immune dysregulation, polyendocrinopathy, enteropathy, X-linked syndrome (IPEX) is caused by mutations of FOXP3. *Nat. Genet.* 2001. 27: 20-21.
[27] Yamanouchi, J., Rainbow, D., Serra, P., Howlett, S., Hunter, K., Garner, V. E., Gonzalez-Munoz, A., Clark, J., Veijola, R., Cubbon, R., Chen, S. L., Rosa, R., Cumiskey, A. M., Serreze, D. V., Gregory, S., Rogers, J., Lyons, P. A., Healy, B., Smink, L. J., Todd, J. A., Peterson, L. B., Wicker, L. S. and Santamaria, P., Interleukin-2 gene variation impairs

regulatory T cell function and causes autoimmunity. *Nat. Genet.* 2007. 39: 329-337.
[28] Kamanaka, M., Rainbow, D., Schuster-Gossler, K., Eynon, E. E., Chervonsky, A. V., Wicker, L. S. and Flavell, R. A., Amino acid polymorphisms altering the glycosylation of IL-2 do not protect from type 1 diabetes in the NOD mouse. *Proc. Natl. Acad. Sci. U. S. A.* 2009. 106: 11236-11240.
[29] Anderson, A. C., Chandwaskar, R., Lee, D. H. and Kuchroo, V. K., Cutting Edge: The Idd3 Genetic Interval Determines Regulatory T Cell Function through CD11b+CD11c- APC. *J. Immunol.* 2008. 181: 7449-7452.
[30] Sgouroudis, E., Albanese, A. and Piccirillo, C. A., Impact of protective IL-2 allelic variants on CD4+ Foxp3+ regulatory T cell function in situ and resistance to autoimmune diabetes in NOD mice. *J. Immunol.* 2008. 181: 6283-6292.
[31] Tang, Q., Adams, J. Y., Penaranda, C., Melli, K., Piaggio, E., Sgouroudis, E., Piccirillo, C. A., Salomon, B. L. and Bluestone, J. A., Central Role of Defective Interleukin-2 Production in the Triggering of Islet Autoimmune Destruction. *Immunity.* 2008.
[32] McGuire, H. M., Vogelzang, A., Hill, N., Flodstrom-Tullberg, M., Sprent, J. and King, C., Loss of parity between IL-2 and IL-21 in the NOD Idd3 locus. *Proc. Natl. Acad. Sci. U. S. A.* 2009.
[33] Lambolez, F., Kronenberg, M. and Cheroutre, H., Thymic differentiation of TCR alpha beta(+) CD8 alpha alpha(+) IELs. *Immunol. Rev.* 2007. 215: 178-188.
[34] Ford, M. S., Chen, W., Wong, S., Li, C., Vanama, R., Elford, A. R., Asa, S. L., Ohashi, P. S. and Zhang, L., Peptide-activated double-negative T cells can prevent autoimmune type-1 diabetes development. *Eur. J. Immunol.* 2007. 37: 2234-2241.
[35] Dugas, V., Beauchamp, C., Chabot-Roy, G., Hillhouse, E. E. and Lesage, S., Implication of the CD47 pathway in autoimmune diabetes. *J. Autoimmun.*
[36] Gardner, J. M., Devoss, J. J., Friedman, R. S., Wong, D. J., Tan, Y. X., Zhou, X., Johannes, K. P., Su, M. A., Chang, H. Y., Krummel, M. F. and Anderson, M. S., Deletional tolerance mediated by extrathymic Aire-expressing cells. *Science.* 2008. 321: 843-847.
[37] Lee, J. W., Epardaud, M., Sun, J., Becker, J. E., Cheng, A. C., Yonekura, A. R., Heath, J. K. and Turley, S. J., Peripheral antigen display by lymph

node stroma promotes T cell tolerance to intestinal self. *Nat. Immunol.* 2007. 8: 181-190.

[38] Linsley, P. S. and Ledbetter, J. A., The role of the CD28 receptor during T cell responses to antigen. *Annu. Rev. Immunol.* 1993. 11: 191-212.

[39] Lesage, S. and Goodnow, C. C., Organ-specific autoimmune disease: a deficiency of tolerogenic stimulation. *J. Exp. Med.* 2001. 194: F31-36.

[40] Salomon, B., Lenschow, D. J., Rhee, L., Ashourian, N., Singh, B., Sharpe, A. and Bluestone, J. A., B7/CD28 costimulation is essential for the homeostasis of the CD4+CD25+ immunoregulatory T cells that control autoimmune diabetes. *Immunity.* 2000. 12: 431-440.

[41] Zeng, M., Guinet, E. and Nouri-Shirazi, M., B7-1 and B7-2 differentially control peripheral homeostasis of CD4(+)CD25(+)Foxp3(+) regulatory T cells. *Transpl. Immunol.* 2009. 20: 171-179.

[42] Greenwald, R. J., Freeman, G. J. and Sharpe, A. H., The B7 family revisited. *Annu. Rev. Immunol.* 2005. 23: 515-548.

[43] Greenwald, R. J., Boussiotis, V. A., Lorsbach, R. B., Abbas, A. K. and Sharpe, A. H., CTLA-4 regulates induction of anergy in vivo. *Immunity.* 2001. 14: 145-155.

[44] Wing, K., Onishi, Y., Prieto-Martin, P., Yamaguchi, T., Miyara, M., Fehervari, Z., Nomura, T. and Sakaguchi, S., CTLA-4 control over Foxp3+ regulatory T cell function. *Science.* 2008. 322: 271-275.

[45] Chambers, C. A., Cado, D., Truong, T. and Allison, J. P., Thymocyte development is normal in CTLA-4-deficient mice. *Proc. Natl. Acad. Sci. U. S. A.* 1997. 94: 9296-9301.

[46] Tivol, E. A., Borriello, F., Schweitzer, A. N., Lynch, W. P., Bluestone, J. A. and Sharpe, A. H., Loss of CTLA-4 leads to massive lymphoproliferation and fatal multiorgan tissue destruction, revealing a critical negative regulatory role of CTLA-4. *Immunity.* 1995. 3: 541-547.

[47] Hill, N. J., Lyons, P. A., Armitage, N., Todd, J. A., Wicker, L. S. and Peterson, L. B., NOD Idd5 locus controls insulitis and diabetes and overlaps the orthologous CTLA4/IDDM12 and NRAMP1 loci in humans. *Diabetes.* 2000. 49: 1744-1747.

[48] Ueda, H., Howson, J. M., Esposito, L., Heward, J., Snook, H., Chamberlain, G., Rainbow, D. B., Hunter, K. M., Smith, A. N., Di Genova, G., Herr, M. H., Dahlman, I., Payne, F., Smyth, D., Lowe, C., Twells, R. C., Howlett, S., Healy, B., Nutland, S., Rance, H. E., Everett, V., Smink, L. J., Lam, A. C., Cordell, H. J., Walker, N. M., Bordin, C., Hulme, J., Motzo, C., Cucca, F., Hess, J. F., Metzker, M. L., Rogers, J., Gregory, S., Allahabadia, A., Nithiyananthan, R., Tuomilehto-Wolf, E.,

Tuomilehto, J., Bingley, P., Gillespie, K. M., Undlien, D. E., Ronningen, K. S., Guja, C., Ionescu-Tirgoviste, C., Savage, D. A., Maxwell, A. P., Carson, D. J., Patterson, C. C., Franklyn, J. A., Clayton, D. G., Peterson, L. B., Wicker, L. S., Todd, J. A. and Gough, S. C., Association of the T-cell regulatory gene CTLA4 with susceptibility to autoimmune disease. *Nature.* 2003. 423: 506-511.

[49] Maier, L. M. and Hafler, D. A., Autoimmunity risk alleles in costimulation pathways. *Immunol. Rev.* 2009. 229: 322-336.

[50] Vijayakrishnan, L., Slavik, J. M., Illes, Z., Greenwald, R. J., Rainbow, D., Greve, B., Peterson, L. B., Hafler, D. A., Freeman, G. J., Sharpe, A. H., Wicker, L. S. and Kuchroo, V. K., An autoimmune disease-associated CTLA-4 splice variant lacking the B7 binding domain signals negatively in T cells. *Immunity.* 2004. 20: 563-575.

[51] Anjos, S. M. and Polychronakos, C., Functional evaluation of the autoimmunity-associated CTLA4 gene: The effect of the (AT) repeat in the 3'untranslated region (UTR). *J. Autoimmun.* 2006.

[52] Chen, Z., Stockton, J., Mathis, D. and Benoist, C., Modeling CTLA4-linked autoimmunity with RNA interference in mice. *Proc. Natl. Acad. Sci. U. S. A.* 2006. 103: 16400-16405.

[53] Araki, M., Chung, D., Liu, S., Rainbow, D. B., Chamberlain, G., Garner, V., Hunter, K. M., Vijayakrishnan, L., Peterson, L. B., Oukka, M., Sharpe, A. H., Sobel, R., Kuchroo, V. K. and Wicker, L. S., Genetic evidence that the differential expression of the ligand-independent isoform of CTLA-4 is the molecular basis of the Idd5.1 type 1 diabetes region in nonobese diabetic mice. *J. Immunol.* 2009. 183: 5146-5157.

[54] Fife, B. T. and Bluestone, J. A., Control of peripheral T-cell tolerance and autoimmunity via the CTLA-4 and PD-1 pathways. *Immunol. Rev.* 2008. 224: 166-182.

[55] Nishimura, H., Okazaki, T., Tanaka, Y., Nakatani, K., Hara, M., Matsumori, A., Sasayama, S., Mizoguchi, A., Hiai, H., Minato, N. and Honjo, T., Autoimmune dilated cardiomyopathy in PD-1 receptor-deficient mice. *Science.* 2001. 291: 319-322.

[56] Nishimura, H., Nose, M., Hiai, H., Minato, N. and Honjo, T., Development of lupus-like autoimmune diseases by disruption of the PD-1 gene encoding an ITIM motif-carrying immunoreceptor. *Immunity.* 1999. 11: 141-151.

[57] Steinman, L., A brief history of T(H)17, the first major revision in the T(H)1/T(H)2 hypothesis of T cell-mediated tissue damage. *Nat. Med.* 2007. 13: 139-145.

[58] Weaver, C. T., Hatton, R. D., Mangan, P. R. and Harrington, L. E., IL-17 family cytokines and the expanding diversity of effector T cell lineages. *Annu. Rev. Immunol.* 2007. 25: 821-852.
[59] Kroenke, M. A., Carlson, T. J., Andjelkovic, A. V. and Segal, B. M., IL-12- and IL-23-modulated T cells induce distinct types of EAE based on histology, CNS chemokine profile, and response to cytokine inhibition. *J. Exp. Med.* 2008. 205: 1535-1541.
[60] Ogura, H., Murakami, M., Okuyama, Y., Tsuruoka, M., Kitabayashi, C., Kanamoto, M., Nishihara, M., Iwakura, Y. and Hirano, T., Interleukin-17 promotes autoimmunity by triggering a positive-feedback loop via interleukin-6 induction. *Immunity.* 2008. 29: 628-636.
[61] Rabinovitch, A., Suarez-Pinzon, W. L., Sorensen, O., Bleackley, R. C. and Power, R. F., IFN-gamma gene expression in pancreatic islet-infiltrating mononuclear cells correlates with autoimmune diabetes in nonobese diabetic mice. *J. Immunol.* 1995. 154: 4874-4882.
[62] Korn, T., Bettelli, E., Oukka, M. and Kuchroo, V. K., IL-17 and Th17 Cells. *Annu. Rev. Immunol.* 2009.
[63] Kleinschek, M. A., Owyang, A. M., Joyce-Shaikh, B., Langrish, C. L., Chen, Y., Gorman, D. M., Blumenschein, W. M., McClanahan, T., Brombacher, F., Hurst, S. D., Kastelein, R. A. and Cua, D. J., IL-25 regulates Th17 function in autoimmune inflammation. *J. Exp. Med.* 2007. 204: 161-170.
[64] Cua, D. J., Sherlock, J., Chen, Y., Murphy, C. A., Joyce, B., Seymour, B., Lucian, L., To, W., Kwan, S., Churakova, T., Zurawski, S., Wiekowski, M., Lira, S. A., Gorman, D., Kastelein, R. A. and Sedgwick, J. D., Interleukin-23 rather than interleukin-12 is the critical cytokine for autoimmune inflammation of the brain. *Nature.* 2003. 421: 744-748.
[65] Adorini, L., Interleukin 12 and autoimmune diabetes. *Nat. Genet.* 2001. 27: 131-132.
[66] Zhou, L., Ivanov, II, Spolski, R., Min, R., Shenderov, K., Egawa, T., Levy, D. E., Leonard, W. J. and Littman, D. R., IL-6 programs T(H)-17 cell differentiation by promoting sequential engagement of the IL-21 and IL-23 pathways. *Nat. Immunol.* 2007. 8: 967-974.
[67] Huber, M., Brustle, A., Reinhard, K., Guralnik, A., Walter, G., Mahiny, A., von Low, E. and Lohoff, M., IRF4 is essential for IL-21-mediated induction, amplification, and stabilization of the Th17 phenotype. *Proc. Natl. Acad. Sci. U. S. A.* 2008. 105: 20846-20851.
[68] Simpson, P. B., Mistry, M. S., Maki, R. A., Yang, W., Schwarz, D. A., Johnson, E. B., Lio, F. M. and Alleva, D. G., Cuttine edge: diabetes-

associated quantitative trait locus, Idd4, is responsible for the IL-12p40 overexpression defect in nonobese diabetic (NOD) mice. *J. Immunol.* 2003. 171: 3333-3337.

[69] Spolski, R., Kashyap, M., Robinson, C., Yu, Z. and Leonard, W. J., IL-21 signaling is critical for the development of type I diabetes in the NOD mouse. *Proc. Natl. Acad. Sci. U. S. A.* 2008.

[70] Oppmann, B., Lesley, R., Blom, B., Timans, J. C., Xu, Y., Hunte, B., Vega, F., Yu, N., Wang, J., Singh, K., Zonin, F., Vaisberg, E., Churakova, T., Liu, M., Gorman, D., Wagner, J., Zurawski, S., Liu, Y., Abrams, J. S., Moore, K. W., Rennick, D., de Waal-Malefyt, R., Hannum, C., Bazan, J. F. and Kastelein, R. A., Novel p19 protein engages IL-12p40 to form a cytokine, IL-23, with biological activities similar as well as distinct from IL-12. *Immunity.* 2000. 13: 715-725.

[71] Elsaesser, H., Sauer, K. and Brooks, D. G., IL-21 is required to control chronic viral infection. *Science.* 2009. 324: 1569-1572.

[72] Frohlich, A., Kisielow, J., Schmitz, I., Freigang, S., Shamshiev, A. T., Weber, J., Marsland, B. J., Oxenius, A. and Kopf, M., IL-21R on T cells is critical for sustained functionality and control of chronic viral infection. *Science.* 2009. 324: 1576-1580.

[73] Yi, J. S., Du, M. and Zajac, A. J., A vital role for interleukin-21 in the control of a chronic viral infection. *Science.* 2009. 324: 1572-1576.

[74] Sutherland, A. P., Van Belle, T., Wurster, A. L., Suto, A., Michaud, M., Zhang, D., Grusby, M. J. and von Herrath, M., Interleukin-21 is required for the development of type 1 diabetes in NOD mice. *Diabetes.* 2009. 58: 1144-1155.

Chapter 3

B CELLS

Erin E. Hillhouse
University of Montreal, Department of Microbiology
and Immunology, Montreal, Quebec, Canada.
Maisonneuve-Rosemont Hospital Research Center, Cellular
Immunogenetics Unit, Montreal, Quebec, Canada.

INTRODUCTION

B lymphocytes are an important part of our adaptive immune system. The principal functions of B cells are to act as APCs, produce antibodies, and develop into memory B cells after activation. Activation of the B cell occurs when the B cell receptor (BCR), which is a membrane-bound immunoglobulin, binds with sufficient affinity to extracellular antigen. Upon activation, the B cell can further differentiate into either a plasma B cell or a memory B cell, both of which will maintain their antigenic-specificity and increase their affinity towards the antigen. Affinity maturation contributes to the enhanced immune response which occurs upon antigen re-encounter.

B CELL TOLERANCE

The BCR itself recognize not only foreign, but also self-antigens. To prevent destructive autoimmune responses, B cells are subject to various immune tolerance mechanisms [1-3]. Indeed, it has been suggested that up to

75% of newly produced B cells carry BCRs that are highly autoreactive [4-6]. Therefore, immune tolerance must be tightly regulated. The first mechanisms of B cell immune tolerance take place as B cells are maturing in the bone marrow and are thus collectively referred to as central tolerance. Indeed, if immature B cells recognize self-antigens with high avidity, they are eliminated by a process known as clonal deletion, which results in apoptosis. Yet, potentially autoreactive immature B cells that recognize self-antigens are not always eliminated. For one, surface IgM expression may be down-regulated sufficiently to allow maturation of the B cell. Secondly, intracellular signaling pathways may be altered to decrease their potential to respond towards self-antigen. This process leads to B cell anergy and allows maturation of unresponsive B cells. Finally, central tolerance mechanisms are not fail-safe allowing some autoreactive B cells that recognize low avidity self-antigens to survive and make their way into the periphery. Here, peripheral tolerance mechanisms will further restrict autoreactive B cells through clonal deletion, anergy, receptor editing and extrinsic suppression [7]. Nevertheless, a defect in any of the various mechanisms involved in immune tolerance would increase the pool of autoreactive B cells and facilitate the progression of autoimmune diseases.

AUTOREACTIVE B CELL ACTIVATION

For autoimmune disease progression, it is not sufficient to carry a high number of potentially autoreactive B cells; these cells must recognize their cognate antigen and be fully activated. Cytokines play an important role in the activation of autoreactive B cells. Type I interferon (IFN) has both direct and indirect effects on B cells [8-11]. Type I IFN can indirectly enhance B cell responses through the activation of DCs, which will then secrete cytokines, such as IFN and B cell activating factor (BAFF), which can then directly stimulate B cell responses [10, 11]. BAFF is a member of the tumour necrosis factor (TNF) family that induces B cell proliferation and promotes B cell survival [12]. In fact, peripheral B cell survival depends on the ability of the cells to compete for BAFF [13]. Under normal circumstances, autoreactive B cells will die in the periphery due to the limited availability of BAFF paired with their reduced responsiveness to this cytokine [14]. However, elevated levels of BAFF are often characteristic of B cell-induced autoimmune diseases [12] where increased levels of this cytokine will result in the rescue of autoreactive B cells that would have normally been deleted. Therefore, B cell-activating cytokines play an important role in the development of autoimmune diseases since they do not neglect autoreactive B cells of their stimulatory effect.

Toll-like receptors (TLRs) can also activate autoreactive B cells and therefore are directly involved in the break in B cell tolerance. TLRs, part of the pattern recognition receptors (PRR), are expressed by a multitude of cells, including monocytes, macrophages, DC and B cells, and recognize pathogen-associated molecular patterns (PAMPs). Amongst the cells that express TLRs, B cells exhibit a unique status as they also express an antigen-specific receptor, the BCR. In fact, TLR expression is upregulated in B cells after BCR activation [15]. It is the simultaneous activation of TLRs and the BCR on autoreactive B cells that induces their proliferation, up-regulation of co-stimulatory molecules, secretion of pro-inflammatory cytokines and the differentiation into plasma cells that produce high levels of autoantibodies [16]. Consequently, TLR activation has a direct effect on autoreactive B cell activation, but also indirectly activates autoreactive T cells as the up-regulation of co-stimulatory molecules on autoreactive B cells results in more efficient antigen-presentation. More specifically, TLR-activated B cells are known to play an important role in the development of various autoimmune diseases such as arthritis [17], experimental autoimmune encephalomyelitis (EAE) [18], which is a model of MS, as well as T1D [19]. Therefore, TLRs are clearly involved in autoimmune disease development.

A Preventive Role for B Cells

Autoreactive B cells promote autoimmune disease progression by secreting pathogenic autoantibodies and presenting autoantigens to T cells. Yet, B cells can also play an essential role in impeding autoimmune disease development. For instance, IL-10-producing B cells have been suggested to resolve or completely inhibit disease development for EAE, arthritis, chronic intestinal inflammation as well as MS [20-24]. In fact, B cells critically depend on TLR to produce IL-10 in order to suppress inflammation [25]. Therefore, B cells themselves can have diverse affects on the outcome of autoimmunity.

AUTOREACTIVE B CELLS IN DISEASE

Nonetheless, autoreactive B cells clearly play an important role in the development of autoimmunity. Autoreactive B cells promote disease not only by the production of autoantibodies, but also by serving as APCs for autoreactive T cells [16]. More specifically, B cells are known to play a role in the development of several autoimmune diseases, such as RA, SLE, Sjogren's syndrome, autoimmune thyroiditis and others [16]. A major challenge has been to determine what leads to the break in B cell tolerance resulting in disease progression. Defects in B cell tolerance mechanisms lead to increased frequencies of autoreactive B cells in the periphery where the over-expression of B cell-activating cytokines and TLR signalling evidently contribute to disease progression.

B CELLS AND GENETICS

As mentioned above, autoreactive B cells are a part of the normal naïve B cell repertoire in the periphery. However, most autoreactive B cells remain functionally naïve for autoantibody production by differential peripheral checkpoints, such as receptor editing, clonal deletion, and anergy. Therefore, the presence of autoreactive B cells does not always signify disease, which is mediated through the regulation of their activation and function. Nevertheless, the existence of pathogenic autoantibodies is often indicative of a break in B cell tolerance and autoimmune disease development.

Recent studies have significantly advanced our understanding of the mechanisms by which autoreactive B cells escape tolerance. A large number of loci and candidate genes are associated with susceptibility to the development of autoimmune diseases, in particular SLE, which is a multigenic autoimmune disease characterized by the production of autoantibodies due to a breakdown in tolerance [26-30]. Among these, defects in the inhibitory Fc receptor (FcγRIIB), a component of the inhibitory signalling pathway that is important for the maintenance of B cell tolerance, are genetically associated with the development of autoimmunity. Indeed, the partial restoration of FcγRIIB levels on B cells from lupus-prone mouse strains is sufficient to prevent disease development [31]. However, the precise mechanism by which FcγRIIB expression on B cells contributes to B cell tolerance maintenance is still under investigation. Moreover, a Y chromosome-linked "autoimmune accelerator" locus (Yaa), in combination with the FcγRIIB gene, significantly increases the onset and severity of lupus development in non-autoimmune-prone C57BL/6 mice [32]. Interestingly, B cells containing the Yaa locus exhibit increased TLR7 expression, which responds to RNA-related antigen stimulation, resulting in increased B cell sensitivity to RNA-containing self-antigens and their subsequent activation [33]. In addition, TLR7 translocation has shown to accelerate SLE autoimmunity [34]. Thus, both the FcγRIIB gene and Yaa locus have been associated with SLE susceptibility.

Genetic studies have also highlighted Ly108, a glycoprotein expressed by B cells belonging to the signalling lymphocytic activation molecule (SLAM) family, as a lupus susceptibility gene [26]. *Ly108* is located on murine chromosome 1 and is associated with the production of autoantibody to chromatin. Thus, autoreactive B cells with an elevated level of expression of the Ly108.1 isoform escape multiple B cell tolerance mechanisms such as deletion, receptor revision, and anergy induction by tuning down BCR signalling at the immature stage of B cell development. Therefore the *Ly108* gene plays a pivotal role in the regulation of autoreactive B cell checkpoints.

Using a GWAS approach, an association between B-cell scaffold protein with ankyrin repeats 1 (BANK1) and SLE was identified. BANK1 variants affect the regulatory sites and key functional domains of the gene [35], which may contribute to sustain B cell-receptor signalling and B-cell hyperactivity, both of which are characteristic of the disease.

Finally, a GWAS mapped the control of marginal zone (MZ) B cell expansion to a region on chromosome 4, which includes the *Idd11* diabetes susceptibility loci, with a LOD score of 4.4 [36]. Interestingly, MZ B cells are expanded 2- to 3-fold in NOD mice compared with non-diabetic C57BL/6 mice by 3 weeks of age, the time when autoreactive T cells are first activated. This supports the hypothesis that this B cell trait is related to the development of diabetes in the NOD mouse.

CONCLUSION

Altogether, our increased understanding of how autoreactive B cells are activated and regulated has led to the emergence of several therapeutic approaches that focus on the blockade of co-stimulatory signals, the specific targeting of the BCR and the depletion of B cells altogether [37]. Indeed, impressive results have been obtained using rituximab, an antibody to CD20 that specifically depletes B cells [38]. However, as mentioned above, B cells can also prevent autoimmune disease progression and, thus, depletion of B cells may not always be beneficial. Consequently, none of these therapies are perfect and they will inevitably affect other aspects of the immune system. Therefore, further investigation is necessary in order to advance our knowledge of immune dysregulation and to enhance the design of autoimmune disease therapies. In the following chapter, the role of another key APC, namely the dendritic cell, and its contribution to autoimmune disease progression is presented.

REFERENCES

[1] Gay, D., Saunders, T., Camper, S. and Weigert, M., Receptor editing: an approach by autoreactive B cells to escape tolerance. *J. Exp. Med.* 1993. 177: 999-1008.

[2] Goodnow, C. C., Crosbie, J., Adelstein, S., Lavoie, T. B., Smith-Gill, S. J., Brink, R. A., Pritchard-Briscoe, H., Wotherspoon, J. S., Loblay, R. H., Raphael, K. and et al., Altered immunoglobulin expression and functional silencing of self-reactive B lymphocytes in transgenic mice. *Nature.* 1988. 334: 676-682.

[3] Nemazee, D. A. and Burki, K., Clonal deletion of B lymphocytes in a transgenic mouse bearing anti-MHC class I antibody genes. *Nature.* 1989. 337: 562-566.

[4] Merrell, K. T., Benschop, R. J., Gauld, S. B., Aviszus, K., Decote-Ricardo, D., Wysocki, L. J. and Cambier, J. C., Identification of anergic B cells within a wild-type repertoire. *Immunity.* 2006. 25: 953-962.

[5] Wardemann, H., Yurasov, S., Schaefer, A., Young, J. W., Meffre, E. and Nussenzweig, M. C., Predominant autoantibody production by early human B cell precursors. *Science.* 2003. 301: 1374-1377.

[6] Novobrantseva, T., Xu, S., Tan, J. E., Maruyama, M., Schwers, S., Pelanda, R. and Lam, K. P., Stochastic pairing of Ig heavy and light chains frequently generates B cell antigen receptors that are subject to editing in vivo. *Int. Immunol.* 2005. 17: 343-350.

[7] Goodnow, C. C., Sprent, J., Fazekas de St Groth, B. and Vinuesa, C. G., Cellular and genetic mechanisms of self tolerance and autoimmunity. *Nature.* 2005. 435: 590-597.

[8] Braun, D., Caramalho, I. and Demengeot, J., IFN-alpha/beta enhances BCR-dependent B cell responses. *Int. Immunol.* 2002. 14: 411-419.

[9] Coro, E. S., Chang, W. L. and Baumgarth, N., Type I IFN receptor signals directly stimulate local B cells early following influenza virus infection. *J. Immunol.* 2006. 176: 4343-4351.

[10] Jego, G., Palucka, A. K., Blanck, J. P., Chalouni, C., Pascual, V. and Banchereau, J., Plasmacytoid dendritic cells induce plasma cell differentiation through type I interferon and interleukin 6. *Immunity.* 2003. 19: 225-234.

[11] Le Bon, A., Schiavoni, G., D'Agostino, G., Gresser, I., Belardelli, F. and Tough, D. F., Type i interferons potently enhance humoral immunity and can promote isotype switching by stimulating dendritic cells in vivo. *Immunity.* 2001. 14: 461-470.

[12] Mackay, F. and Schneider, P., Cracking the BAFF code. *Nat. Rev. Immunol.* 2009. 9: 491-502.

[13] Stadanlick, J. E. and Cancro, M. P., BAFF and the plasticity of peripheral B cell tolerance. *Curr. Opin. Immunol.* 2008. 20: 158-161.

[14] Brink, R., Regulation of B cell self-tolerance by BAFF. *Semin. Immunol.* 2006. 18: 276-283.

[15] Bernasconi, N. L., Onai, N. and Lanzavecchia, A., A role for Toll-like receptors in acquired immunity: up-regulation of TLR9 by BCR triggering in naive B cells and constitutive expression in memory B cells. *Blood.* 2003. 101: 4500-4504.

[16] Meyer-Bahlburg, A. and Rawlings, D. J., B cell autonomous TLR signaling and autoimmunity. *Autoimmun. Rev.* 2008. 7: 313-316.

[17] Deng, G. M., Nilsson, I. M., Verdrengh, M., Collins, L. V. and Tarkowski, A., Intra-articularly localized bacterial DNA containing CpG motifs induces arthritis. *Nat. Med.* 1999. 5: 702-705.

[18] Segal, B. M., Chang, J. T. and Shevach, E. M., CpG oligonucleotides are potent adjuvants for the activation of autoreactive encephalitogenic T cells in vivo. *J. Immunol.* 2000. 164: 5683-5688.

[19] Lang, K. S., Recher, M., Junt, T., Navarini, A. A., Harris, N. L., Freigang, S., Odermatt, B., Conrad, C., Ittner, L. M., Bauer, S., Luther, S. A., Uematsu, S., Akira, S., Hengartner, H. and Zinkernagel, R. M., Toll-like receptor engagement converts T-cell autoreactivity into overt autoimmune disease. *Nat. Med.* 2005. 11: 138-145.

[20] Fillatreau, S., Sweenie, C. H., McGeachy, M. J., Gray, D. and Anderton, S. M., B cells regulate autoimmunity by provision of IL-10. *Nat. Immunol.* 2002. 3: 944-950.

[21] Mauri, C., Gray, D., Mushtaq, N. and Londei, M., Prevention of arthritis by interleukin 10-producing B cells. *J. Exp. Med.* 2003. 197: 489-501.

[22] Mizoguchi, A., Mizoguchi, E., Takedatsu, H., Blumberg, R. S. and Bhan, A. K., Chronic intestinal inflammatory condition generates IL-10-producing regulatory B cell subset characterized by CD1d upregulation. *Immunity.* 2002. 16: 219-230.
[23] Duddy, M. E., Alter, A. and Bar-Or, A., Distinct profiles of human B cell effector cytokines: a role in immune regulation? *J. Immunol.* 2004. 172: 3422-3427.
[24] Duddy, M., Niino, M., Adatia, F., Hebert, S., Freedman, M., Atkins, H., Kim, H. J. and Bar-Or, A., Distinct effector cytokine profiles of memory and naive human B cell subsets and implication in multiple sclerosis. *J. Immunol.* 2007. 178: 6092-6099.
[25] Lampropoulou, V., Hoehlig, K., Roch, T., Neves, P., Calderon Gomez, E., Sweenie, C. H., Hao, Y., Freitas, A. A., Steinhoff, U., Anderton, S. M. and Fillatreau, S., TLR-activated B cells suppress T cell-mediated autoimmunity. *J. Immunol.* 2008. 180: 4763-4773.
[26] Kumar, K. R., Li, L., Yan, M., Bhaskarabhatla, M., Mobley, A. B., Nguyen, C., Mooney, J. M., Schatzle, J. D., Wakeland, E. K. and Mohan, C., Regulation of B cell tolerance by the lupus susceptibility gene Ly108. *Science.* 2006. 312: 1665-1669.
[27] Morel, L., Croker, B. P., Blenman, K. R., Mohan, C., Huang, G., Gilkeson, G. and Wakeland, E. K., Genetic reconstitution of systemic lupus erythematosus immunopathology with polycongenic murine strains. *Proc. Natl. Acad. Sci. U. S. A.* 2000. 97: 6670-6675.
[28] Morel, L. and Wakeland, E. K., Lessons from the NZM2410 model and related strains. *Int. Rev. Immunol.* 2000. 19: 423-446.
[29] Vyse, T. J. and Kotzin, B. L., Genetic susceptibility to systemic lupus erythematosus. *Annu. Rev. Immunol.* 1998. 16: 261-292.
[30] Vyse, T. J., Rozzo, S. J., Drake, C. G., Appel, V. B., Lemeur, M., Izui, S., Palmer, E. and Kotzin, B. L., Contributions of Ea(z) and Eb(z) MHC genes to lupus susceptibility in New Zealand mice. *J. Immunol.* 1998. 160: 2757-2766.
[31] McGaha, T. L., Sorrentino, B. and Ravetch, J. V., Restoration of tolerance in lupus by targeted inhibitory receptor expression. *Science.* 2005. 307: 590-593.
[32] Bolland, S., Yim, Y. S., Tus, K., Wakeland, E. K. and Ravetch, J. V., Genetic modifiers of systemic lupus erythematosus in FcgammaRIIB(-/-) mice. *J Exp Med* 2002. 195: 1167-1174.
[33] Pisitkun, P., Deane, J. A., Difilippantonio, M. J., Tarasenko, T., Satterthwaite, A. B. and Bolland, S., Autoreactive B cell responses to

RNA-related antigens due to TLR7 gene duplication. *Science.* 2006. 312: 1669-1672.

[34] Subramanian, S., Tus, K., Li, Q. Z., Wang, A., Tian, X. H., Zhou, J., Liang, C., Bartov, G., McDaniel, L. D., Zhou, X. J., Schultz, R. A. and Wakeland, E. K., A Tlr7 translocation accelerates systemic autoimmunity in murine lupus. *Proc. Natl. Acad. Sci. U. S. A.* 2006. 103: 9970-9975.

[35] Kozyrev, S. V., Abelson, A. K., Wojcik, J., Zaghlool, A., Linga Reddy, M. V., Sanchez, E., Gunnarsson, I., Svenungsson, E., Sturfelt, G., Jonsen, A., Truedsson, L., Pons-Estel, B. A., Witte, T., D'Alfonso, S., Barizzone, N., Danieli, M. G., Gutierrez, C., Suarez, A., Junker, P., Laustrup, H., Gonzalez-Escribano, M. F., Martin, J., Abderrahim, H. and Alarcon-Riquelme, M. E., Functional variants in the B-cell gene BANK1 are associated with systemic lupus erythematosus. *Nat. Genet.* 2008. 40: 211-216.

[36] Rolf, J., Motta, V., Duarte, N., Lundholm, M., Berntman, E., Bergman, M. L., Sorokin, L., Cardell, S. L. and Holmberg, D., The enlarged population of marginal zone/CD1d(high) B lymphocytes in nonobese diabetic mice maps to diabetes susceptibility region Idd11. *J. Immunol.* 2005. 174: 4821-4827.

[37] Blank, M. and Shoenfeld, Y., B cell targeted therapy in autoimmunity. *J. Autoimmun.* 2007. 28: 62-68.

[38] Perosa, F., Favoino, E., Caragnano, M. A., Prete, M. and Dammacco, F., CD20: a target antigen for immunotherapy of autoimmune diseases. *Autoimmun. Rev.* 2005. 4: 526-531.

Chapter 4

DENDRITIC CELL SUBSETS

Sylvie Lesage, Adam-Nicolas Pelletier and Fanny Guimont-Desrochers

University of Montreal, Department of
Microbiology and Immunology, Montreal, Quebec, Canada.
Maisonneuve-Rosemont Hospital Research Center, Cellular
Immunogenetics Unit, Montreal, Quebec, Canada.

INTRODUCTION

Dendritic cells (DCs), which were described quite recently relative to other immune cell types [1-5], compose approximately 1% of the immune cells found in the spleen. Despite their limited proportions, they entice immunologists due to their prominent antigen presenting potential [6]. Indeed, they are considered as the professional APC with the highest proficiency for activating naïve T cells, which places them at the bridge between innate and adaptive immunity. This central position within the immune response suggests that the modulation of this cell type may provide new therapeutic approaches in cancer, autoimmunity and vaccination. Consequently, DCs have been extensively studied since their initial description and are now known to include many distinct subsets with unique phenotypes that carry out a multitude of immune functions.

Apart from their role in activating the adaptive arm of the immune system, DCs significantly contribute to immune tolerance mechanisms. Indeed, DCs clearly impact both central and peripheral induction of T cell tolerance. Thus, a better understanding of the underlying mechanism of tolerance induction may provide clues regarding how defects in this pathway may favour the development of autoimmunity.

T CELL TOLERANCE AS MEDIATED BY DENDRITIC CELLS

Central tolerance is mostly mediated by the process of negative selection of potentially autoreactive clones. DCs contribute to this process by presenting self-antigens to T cells [7]. Thymic dendritic cell subsets include $CD8\alpha^+CD172a^-$ DC, $CD8\alpha^-CD172a^+$ DC, and plasmacytoid DC (pDC) [8, 9], where the role of pDC in thymic tolerance has yet to be examined. The $CD8\alpha^+CD172a^-$ DCs differentiate from thymic precursors while the $CD8\alpha^-CD172a^+$ DCs recirculate from the periphery [10, 11]. Therefore, $CD8\alpha^+CD172a^-$ DCs present thymic self-antigens while $CD8\alpha^-CD172a^+$ DCs present peripheral self-antigens to thymocytes. Thus, together, these DC subsets allow for the efficient deletion of thymocytes expressing a potentially autoreactive TCR. Most recently, it has been suggested that $CD8\alpha^-CD172a^+$ DCs also contribute to T cell tolerance processes by promoting the differentiation of Tregs [11, 12]. As tDCs play a key role in mediating central tolerance, defects in thymic subsets should, thus, have dire consequences and promote autoimmune progression. However, negative selection processes are not affected in mice deficient for CD47, the counter-ligand of CD172a necessary for transmigration of $CD172a^+$ cells [13-17], where the proportion of $CD8\alpha^-CD172a^+$ thymic DCs is significantly reduced [17]. Therefore, additional studies are required to determine the exact contribution of thymic DCs to central tolerance mechanisms.

DCs are also known to participate in peripheral immune tolerance. For instance, increasing the number of DCs in NOD mice completely abrogates autoimmune disease onset [18]. Moreover, ablation of DCs in mice results in the induction of an autoimmune phenotype, demonstrating that the presence of DCs at steady state contribute to immune tolerance [19]. Yet, it should be noted that a fine balance exists between the role of DCs in tolerance induction and immune activation. Indeed, promoting DC survival also favours autoimmune progression [20]. Therefore, understanding how DCs function is crucial for the development of appropriate therapeutic approaches.

SPECIFIC ROLE OF DENDRITIC CELL SUBSETS IN IMMUNE TOLERANCE

In recent years, many DC subsets have been described [21]. In mice, the so-called conventional DC (cDC) expresses high levels of CD11c and can be further segregated into two functionally distinct subsets according to the expression of CD8α, where CD8α+ DCs appear to contribute more extensively to tolerance induction than the CD8α- counterpart. Specifically, the CD8α- DCs have been reported to contribute to the pathogenesis of T1D, where they transport β cell antigens from the islets to the pancreatic lymph node, which promotes autoreactive T cell activation facilitating insulitis development [22]. Moreover, specific ablation of CD8α- DCs results in the absence of insulitis and diabetes [23]. However, these results should be interpreted with caution, as CD8α- DCs define two functionally distinct subsets, namely monocyte-derived DCs, which arise in response to inflammation, or a steady state population, which exhibits low levels of co-stimulatory molecules. Clear phenotypic differences between these two subsets have yet to be resolved and, thus, preclude their distinction particularly in an inflammatory context where the inflammatory DC subset predominates. In contrast, the CD8α+ DCs contribute to tolerance induction. In the spleen, CD8α+ DCs specifically express the DEC-205 endocytic receptor. Anti-DEC-205 antibodies directly coupled to antigen can be used to efficiently target CD8α+ DCs *in vivo* without activating DCs. Using this strategy, it was demonstrated that CD8α+ DCs specifically induce T cell tolerance [24, 25]. Interestingly, the lymphoid cDC subset has recently been divided into 2 new subsets in the spleen depending on the expression of the CD103 integrin [26]. The CD103[+] subset has been shown to induce tolerance, as it exhibits an increased potential of cross-presentation relative to the CD103[-] counterpart [26]. Indeed, the ability of CD8α+ DCs to cross-present antigen on MHC class I, which is essential for the tolerization of autoreactive CD8 T cells [27], can now be entirely attributed to the CD103+ subset. Finally, deficiencies in CD8α+ or CD8α- DC subsets by genetic ablation of various transcription factors, such as RelB, IRF-2, IRF-4, IRF8, TRAF6 and PU.1, have been reported to favour autoimmune pathologies [28-35]. Yet, these transcription factors do not exclusively affect the differentiation of these DC subsets, thus, more work is required to determine the specific contribution of DC subset deletion to promoting inflammatory responses and contributing to autoimmune progression.

Although the conventional DC subsets have been more extensively characterized, other DC subsets are emerging as important players in either tolerance or activation mechanisms. One such subset would be the CD11c^{low} B220$^+$ PDCA-1$^+$ pDCs [23]. They are generally known for their great capacity to secrete type I IFN in response to viral infections and tumours. However, pDCs express low levels of MHC class II, a characteristic associated with CD4 T cell tolerance induction [36]. Moreover, pDCs have recently been shown to induce the generation of CD4$^+$CD25$^+$ regulatory T cells [37]. Finally, elimination of pDCs accelerates insulitis onset and diabetes progression [23]. Together, these results suggest that pDCs are important players in preventing autoimmune disease progression.

Recently, a new DC subset named interferon-producing killer dendritic cell (IKDC) has been identified (1). This novel cell type shares phenotypic and functional characteristics of natural killer (NK) cells and DCs, as they can produce impressive amounts of IFN-γ and exhibit cytotoxic activity as well as process and present antigen to naïve T cells [38-41]. Because IKDCs are phenotypically similar to pDCs (low levels of MHC and co-stimulatory molecules), which are known to confer tolerance, IKDCs may play a role in tolerance (4-5). Indeed, low IKDC number is associated with autoimmune diabetes susceptibility when comparing autoimmune-diabetes prone and resistant murine models (6). In order to identify the genetic regions regulating their proportion, a linkage analysis using SNPs was performed and showed that the distal arm of chromosome 7 regulated IKDC number. Moreover, NOD.Lc7 congenic mice carry high numbers of IKDCs, thus, confirming that this genetic interval does indeed regulate IKDC number. Interestingly, NOD.Lc7 mice no longer develop diabetes (7), further supporting the association between IKDC number and autoimmune diabetes resistance.

Although the Lc7 interval regulates IKDC number and confers protection from diabetes progression, much more work is needed to provide a direct link between these two phenotypes. Indeed, the Lc7 interval is involved in preventing islet β cell apoptosis [42]. However, the Lc7 interval encodes for more than 500 genes making it difficult to determine which genes are causal to this phenotype. As a result, diabetes resistance may be due to the β cells' increased resistance to apoptosis, increased IKDC number, other yet undiscovered phenotypes defined by Lc7, or a combination of the effects of many genes within this interval.

Linkage analysis of phenotypic traits results in the identification of genes regulating this trait, but does not directly associate the phenotypic traits with disease susceptibility. Therefore, until the biological function of IKDCs is fully elucidated, these results simply suggest that IKDCs may be involved in tolerance. Hence, further cellular and functional studies are needed to demonstrate a *bona fide* role of the IKDC subset in tolerance. Still, the identification of the particular genes regulating IKDC number on chromosomes 7 may prove useful in defining the contribution of IKDCs to autoimmune diabetes susceptibility.

Whether the subset is beneficial or detrimental to immune tolerance, it is clear that DCs hold a vital importance in immune tolerance. The various mechanisms that modulate the autoimmune response and tolerance induction constitute potential interesting treatment methods. It has been shown in NOD mice that T1D can be prevented upon dendritic cell transfer [43], demonstrating that such treatments are may be achievable in humans. There is, however, a need for further characterization of most DC subsets, whether it be regarding their function, proportion or link to autoimmunity. Furthermore, the recent discovery of IKDCs implies that there might be other unknown subtypes of DCs with unique phenotypes that have yet to be discovered that could help explain current issues.

CONCLUSION

Although DCs are present in low number, they clearly play a predominant role in immune tolerance. However, genetic variants involved in defining DC subsets or function have not yet been underlined. This may be a direct consequence of the multiple DC lineages as well as the rarity of this cell type. Still, the modulation of DC number and function may prove critical in the prevention of autoimmune diseases. In the following chapter, the role of macrophages, the third and last APC type, will be discussed in the context of autoimmune disease development.

REFERENCES

[1] Steinman, R. M. and Cohn, Z. A., Identification of a novel cell type in peripheral lymphoid organs of mice. I. Morphology, quantitation, tissue distribution. *J. Exp. Med.* 1973. 137: 1142-1162.

[2] Steinman, R. M. and Cohn, Z. A., Identification of a novel cell type in peripheral lymphoid organs of mice. II. Functional properties in vitro. *J. Exp. Med.* 1974. 139: 380-397.

[3] Steinman, R. M., Lustig, D. S. and Cohn, Z. A., Identification of a novel cell type in peripheral lymphoid organs of mice. 3. Functional properties in vivo. *J. Exp. Med.* 1974. 139: 1431-1445.

[4] Steinman, R. M., Adams, J. C. and Cohn, Z. A., Identification of a novel cell type in peripheral lymphoid organs of mice. IV. Identification and distribution in mouse spleen. *J. Exp. Med.* 1975. 141: 804-820.

[5] Steinman, R. M., Kaplan, G., Witmer, M. D. and Cohn, Z. A., Identification of a novel cell type in peripheral lymphoid organs of mice. V. Purification of spleen dendritic cells, new surface markers, and maintenance in vitro. *J. Exp. Med.* 1979. 149: 1-16.

[6] Steinman, R. M., Gutchinov, B., Witmer, M. D. and Nussenzweig, M. C., Dendritic cells are the principal stimulators of the primary mixed leukocyte reaction in mice. *J. Exp. Med.* 1983. 157: 613-627.

[7] Goldschneider, I. and Cone, R. E., A central role for peripheral dendritic cells in the induction of acquired thymic tolerance. *Trends Immunol.* 2003. 24: 77-81.

[8] Vremec, D., Pooley, J., Hochrein, H., Wu, L. and Shortman, K., CD4 and CD8 expression by dendritic cell subtypes in mouse thymus and spleen. *J. Immunol.* 2000. 164: 2978-2986.

[9] Lahoud, M. H., Proietto, A. I., Gartlan, K. H., Kitsoulis, S., Curtis, J., Wettenhall, J., Sofi, M., Daunt, C., O'Keeffe, M., Caminschi, I., Satterley, K., Rizzitelli, A., Schnorrer, P., Hinohara, A., Yamaguchi, Y., Wu, L., Smyth, G., Handman, E., Shortman, K. and Wright, M. D., Signal regulatory protein molecules are differentially expressed by CD8- dendritic cells. *J. Immunol.* 2006. 177: 372-382.

[10] Donskoy, E. and Goldschneider, I., Two developmentally distinct populations of dendritic cells inhabit the adult mouse thymus: demonstration by differential importation of hematogenous precursors under steady state conditions. *J. Immunol.* 2003. 170: 3514-3521.

[11] Proietto, A. I., van Dommelen, S. and Wu, L., The impact of circulating dendritic cells on the development and differentiation of thymocytes. *Immunol. Cell Biol.* 2009. 87: 39-45.

[12] Proietto, A. I., van Dommelen, S., Zhou, P., Rizzitelli, A., D'Amico, A., Steptoe, R. J., Naik, S. H., Lahoud, M. H., Liu, Y., Zheng, P., Shortman, K. and Wu, L., Dendritic cells in the thymus contribute to T-regulatory cell induction. *Proc. Natl. Acad. Sci. U. S. A.* 2008. 105: 19869-19874.

[13] Lindberg, F. P., Bullard, D. C., Caver, T. E., Gresham, H. D., Beaudet, A. L. and Brown, E. J., Decreased resistance to bacterial infection and granulocyte defects in IAP-deficient mice. *Science.* 1996. 274: 795-798.
[14] Liu, Y., Buhring, H. J., Zen, K., Burst, S. L., Schnell, F. J., Williams, I. R. and Parkos, C. A., Signal regulatory protein (SIRPalpha), a cellular ligand for CD47, regulates neutrophil transmigration. *J. Biol. Chem.* 2002. 277: 10028-10036.
[15] Hagnerud, S., Manna, P. P., Cella, M., Stenberg, A., Frazier, W. A., Colonna, M. and Oldenborg, P. A., Deficit of CD47 Results in a Defect of Marginal Zone Dendritic Cells, Blunted Immune Response to Particulate Antigen and Impairment of Skin Dendritic Cell Migration. *J. Immunol.* 2006. 176: 5772-5778.
[16] Van, V. Q., Lesage, S., Bouguermouh, S., Gautier, P., Rubio, M., Levesque, M., Nguyen, S., Galibert, L. and Sarfati, M., Expression of the self-marker CD47 on dendritic cells governs their trafficking to secondary lymphoid organs. *Embo J.* 2006. 25: 5560-5568.
[17] Guimont-Desrochers, F., Beauchamp, C., Chabot-Roy, G., Dugas, V., Hillhouse, E. E., Dusseault, J., Langlois, G., Gautier-Ethier, P., Darwiche, J., Sarfati, M. and Lesage, S., Absence of CD47 in vivo influences thymic dendritic cell subset proportions but not negative selection of thymocytes. *Int. Immunol.* 2009. 21: 167-177.
[18] O'Keeffe, M., Brodnicki, T. C., Fancke, B., Vremec, D., Morahan, G., Maraskovsky, E., Steptoe, R., Harrison, L. C. and Shortman, K., Fms-like tyrosine kinase 3 ligand administration overcomes a genetically determined dendritic cell deficiency in NOD mice and protects against diabetes development. *Int. Immunol.* 2005. 17: 307-314.
[19] Ohnmacht, C., Pullner, A., King, S. B. S., Drexler, I., Meier, S., Brocker, T. and Voehringer, D., Constitutive ablation of dendritic cells breaks self-tolerance of CD4 T cells and results in spontaneous fatal autoimmunity. *J. Exp. Med.* 2009. 206: 549-559.
[20] Chen, M., Wang, Y. H., Wang, Y., Huang, L., Sandoval, H., Liu, Y. J. and Wang, J., Dendritic cell apoptosis in the maintenance of immune tolerance. *Science.* 2006. 311: 1160-1164.
[21] Shortman, K. and Naik, S. H., Steady-state and inflammatory dendritic-cell development. *Nat. Rev. Immunol.* 2007. 7: 19-30.
[22] Turley, S., Poirot, L., Hattori, M., Benoist, C. and Mathis, D., Physiological beta cell death triggers priming of self-reactive T cells by dendritic cells in a type-1 diabetes model. *J. Exp. Med.* 2003. 198: 1527-1537.

[23] Saxena, V., Ondr, J. K., Magnusen, A. F., Munn, D. H. and Katz, J. D., The countervailing actions of myeloid and plasmacytoid dendritic cells control autoimmune diabetes in the nonobese diabetic mouse. *J. Immunol.* 2007. 179: 5041-5053.

[24] Hawiger, D., Inaba, K., Dorsett, Y., Guo, M., Mahnke, K., Rivera, M., Ravetch, J. V., Steinman, R. M. and Nussenzweig, M. C., Dendritic cells induce peripheral T cell unresponsiveness under steady state conditions in vivo. *J. Exp. Med.* 2001. 194: 769-779.

[25] Bonifaz, L., Bonnyay, D., Mahnke, K., Rivera, M., Nussenzweig, M. C. and Steinman, R. M., Efficient targeting of protein antigen to the dendritic cell receptor DEC-205 in the steady state leads to antigen presentation on major histocompatibility complex class I products and peripheral CD8+ T cell tolerance. *J. Exp. Med.* 2002. 196: 1627-1638.

[26] Qiu, C.-H., Miyake, Y., Kaise, H., Kitamura, H., Ohara, O. and Tanaka, M., Novel Subset of CD8 + Dendritic Cells Localized in the Marginal Zone Is Responsible for Tolerance to Cell-Associated Antigens. *The Journal of Immunology.* 2009. 182: 4127-4136.

[27] Belz, G. T., Behrens, G. M. N., Smith, C. M., Miller, J. F. A. P., Jones, C., Lejon, K., Fathman, C. G., Mueller, S. N., Shortman, K., Carbone, F. R. and Heath, W. R., The CD8alpha(+) dendritic cell is responsible for inducing peripheral self-tolerance to tissue-associated antigens. *J. Exp. Med.* 2002. 196: 1099-1104.

[28] Wu, L., D'Amico, A., Winkel, K. D., Suter, M., Lo, D. and Shortman, K., RelB is essential for the development of myeloid-related CD8alpha-dendritic cells but not of lymphoid-related CD8alpha+ dendritic cells. *Immunity.* 1998. 9: 839-847.

[29] Weih, F., Carrasco, D., Durham, S. K., Barton, D. S., Rizzo, C. A., Ryseck, R. P., Lira, S. A. and Bravo, R., Multiorgan inflammation and hematopoietic abnormalities in mice with a targeted disruption of RelB, a member of the NF-kappa B/Rel family. *Cell.* 1995. 80: 331-340.

[30] Ichikawa, E., Hida, S., Omatsu, Y., Shimoyama, S., Takahara, K., Miyagawa, S., Inaba, K. and Taki, S., Defective development of splenic and epidermal CD4+ dendritic cells in mice deficient for IFN regulatory factor-2. *Proc. Natl. Acad. Sci. U. S. A.* 2004. 101: 3909-3914.

[31] Schiavoni, G., Mattei, F., Sestili, P., Borghi, P., Venditti, M., Morse, H. C., 3rd, Belardelli, F. and Gabriele, L., ICSBP is essential for the development of mouse type I interferon-producing cells and for the generation and activation of CD8alpha(+) dendritic cells. *J. Exp. Med.* 2002. 196: 1415-1425.

[32] Aliberti, J., Schulz, O., Pennington, D. J., Tsujimura, H., Reis e Sousa, C., Ozato, K. and Sher, A., Essential role for ICSBP in the in vivo development of murine CD8alpha + dendritic cells. *Blood.* 2003. 101: 305-310.

[33] Suzuki, S., Honma, K., Matsuyama, T., Suzuki, K., Toriyama, K., Akitoyo, I., Yamamoto, K., Suematsu, T., Nakamura, M., Yui, K. and Kumatori, A., Critical roles of interferon regulatory factor 4 in CD11bhighCD8alpha- dendritic cell development. *Proc. Natl. Acad. Sci. U. S. A.* 2004. 101: 8981-8986.

[34] Tamura, T., Tailor, P., Yamaoka, K., Kong, H. J., Tsujimura, H., O'Shea, J. J., Singh, H. and Ozato, K., IFN regulatory factor-4 and -8 govern dendritic cell subset development and their functional diversity. *J. Immunol.* 2005. 174: 2573-2581.

[35] Kobayashi, T., Walsh, P. T., Walsh, M. C., Speirs, K. M., Chiffoleau, E., King, C. G., Hancock, W. W., Caamano, J. H., Hunter, C. A., Scott, P., Turka, L. A. and Choi, Y., TRAF6 is a critical factor for dendritic cell maturation and development. *Immunity.* 2003. 19: 353-363.

[36] Ochando, J. C., Homma, C., Yang, Y., Hidalgo, A., Garin, A., Tacke, F., Angeli, V., Li, Y., Boros, P., Ding, Y., Jessberger, R., Trinchieri, G., Lira, S. A., Randolph, G. J. and Bromberg, J. S., Alloantigen-presenting plasmacytoid dendritic cells mediate tolerance to vascularized grafts. *Nat. Immunol.* 2006. 7: 652-662.

[37] Chen, W., Liang, X., Peterson, A. J., Munn, D. H. and Blazar, B. R., The indoleamine 2,3-dioxygenase pathway is essential for human plasmacytoid dendritic cell-induced adaptive T regulatory cell generation. *J. Immunol.* 2008. 181: 5396-5404.

[38] Chan, C., Crafton, E., Fan, H., Flook, J., Yoshimura, K., Skarica, M., Brockstedt, D., Dubensky, T., Stins, M., Lanier, L., Pardoll, D. and Housseau, F., Interferon-producing killer dendritic cells provide a link between innate and adaptive immunity. *Nat. Med.* 2006. 12: 207-213.

[39] Himoudi, N., Yan, M., Bouma, G., Morgenstern, D., Wallace, R., Seddon, B., Buddle, J., Eddaoudi, A., Howe, S. J., Cooper, N. and Anderson, J., Migratory and antigen presentation functions of IFN-producing killer dendritic cells. *Cancer Res.* 2009. 69: 6598-6606.

[40] Pletneva, M., Fan, H., Park, J. J., Radojcic, V., Jie, C., Yu, Y., Chan, C., Redwood, A., Pardoll, D. and Housseau, F., IFN-producing killer dendritic cells are antigen-presenting cells endowed with T-cell cross-priming capacity. *Cancer Res.* 2009. 69: 6607-6614.

[41] Terme, M., Mignot, G., Ullrich, E., Bonmort, M., Minard-Colin, V., Jacquet, A., Schultze, J. L., Kroemer, G., Leclerc, C., Chaput, N. and Zitvogel, L., The dendritic cell-like functions of IFN-producing killer dendritic cells reside in the CD11b+ subset and are licensed by tumor cells. *Cancer Res.* 2009. 69: 6590-6597.

[42] Haskins, K., Kench, J., Powers, K., Bradley, B., Pugazhenthi, S., Reusch, J. and McDuffie, M., Role for oxidative stress in the regeneration of islet beta cells? *J. Investig. Med.* 2004. 52: 45-49.

[43] Clare-Salzler, M. J., Brooks, J., Chai, A., Van Herle, K. and Anderson, C., Prevention of diabetes in nonobese diabetic mice by dendritic cell transfer. *J. Clin. Invest.* 1992. 90: 741-748.

Chapter 5

MACROPHAGES

Véronique Dugas[1] and Jean-François Cailhier[2]

[1] University of Montreal, Department of Microbiology and Immunology,
Montreal, Quebec, Canada.
Maisonneuve-Rosemont Hospital Research Center, Cellular
Immunogenetics Unit, Montreal, Quebec, Canada.
[2] University of Montreal, Department of Medecine,
Montreal, Quebec, Canada.
CRCHUM et Institut du Cancer de Montréal,
Pav JA DeSève, Y-4622, Montréal, Québec, Canada.

INTRODUCTION

Macrophages represent a heterogeneous population of mononuclear leukocytes that originate from circulating monocytes to become tissue-resident. However, during the course of infection, monocytes can directly differentiate into activated macrophages and are recruited to sites of inflammation. They recognize pathogens via several receptors specific for antibodies or foreign antigens, such as Fc receptors or TLRs, respectively. Indeed, a variety of PAMPs can trigger macrophage activation, through interaction with numerous extracellular and intracellular PRRs. Upon danger-induced stimulation, macrophages have the ability to kill the pathogens or the infected cells. Moreover, they also present the pathogen-derived antigens to lymphocytes, after which an adaptive immune response ensues.

MACROPHAGES IN TOLERANCE

Other than their roles in cell killing and phagocytosis of pathogens, macrophages are certainly important mediators of tolerance induction. This leukocyte of the innate immune system is involved in the efficient removal of apoptotic cells, a process generally known to contribute to the maintenance of immune tolerance. Indeed, perpetual tissue turnover generates a high number of apoptotic cells, which must be rapidly removed in order to prevent inflammation [1]. Defects in apoptotic cell clearance are thought to be implicated in autoimmune pathologies such as SLE, where autoantibodies specific for intracellular proteins are responsible for inflammation [2]. More particularly, it has been shown that monocyte-derived macrophages from SLE patients display an impaired ability to phagocytose apoptotic cells [3]. Furthermore, removal of apoptotic cells by macrophages, as well as other phagocytes, leads to the secretion of anti-inflammatory cytokines, such as IL-10 and TGF-β, and contributes to the maintenance of immune tolerance [4]. Finally, apoptotic cell uptake allows the presentation of self-antigens by macrophages to T cells in the absence of co-stimulatory molecules, thereby inducing T cell anergy of potentially autoreactive T cells, depending on the absence of other pro-inflammatory or danger signal associated with the apoptotic cells.

In addition to phagocytosis, macrophages can eliminate apoptotic cells through other mechanisms. With dendritic cells, macrophages are responsible for the main production of the C1q complement component, which is known to opsonize apoptotic cells, thereby facilitating their uptake by phagocytes [5]. In addition, C1q binding on apoptotic cells induces TGF-β production by macrophages through enhanced phagocytosis, which in turn facilitates conversion of naïve CD4 T cells into Tregs. C1q in itself can also promote an anti-inflammatory phenotype [6]. Interestingly, C1q-deficient mice have increased tissue apoptotic bodies, and are prone to autoimmunity [7]. Moreover, C1q polymorphisms have been associated with SLE in humans [8, 9].

Other than C1q, the Milk Fat Globule-EGF factor 8 (MFG-E8), a protein first identified in lactating mammary glands and milk fat globules, is also abundantly produced by macrophages following stimulation [10]. The MFG-E8 glycoprotein binds to phosphatidylserines exposed on apoptotic cells, which enhances the uptake by macrophages. Indeed, mice deficient for MFG-E8 present an impaired engulfment of apoptotic cells, as well as an increased predisposition to glomerulonephritis [11, 12]. In humans, genetic polymorphisms of MFG-E8 have also been significantly correlated to SLE susceptibility [10]. Thus, macrophages significantly contribute to induction of immune tolerance, in particular via the clearance of apoptotic cells and the anti-inflammatory, protolerance reprogramming.

MACROPHAGES AND T CELL TOLERANCE

Macrophages can also participate in immune tolerance induction upon interacting with T lymphocytes. On the one hand, macrophages have the capacity to suppress T cell proliferation via the induction of two enzymes involved in amino acid catabolism, indoleamine 2,3-dioxygenase (IDO) and inducible nitric oxide synthase (iNOS) [13]. For instance, IDO is associated with T cell suppression via tryptophan depletion and generation of pro-apoptotic metabolites [14]. Moreover, it has been proposed that NO production is implicated in reducing inflammatory T cell expansion, which is associated with autoimmune diseases [15, 16]. Indeed, EAE remission phases are markedly reduced in mice deficient for *NOS2*, for which NO production is significantly decreased [17]. On the other hand, macrophages are potent inducers of regulatory T cells. For instance, human monocyte-derived macrophages induce the differentiation of IL-10-producing T cells [18]. IL-10 is a potent immunosuppressive cytokine which in turn leads to generalized T cell anergy. Moreover, it has been shown that TGF-β treated macrophages can induce the development of various Treg subsets *in vivo* [19, 20]. Therefore, macrophages significantly contribute to the induction of peripheral T cell tolerance mechanisms.

MACROPHAGES IN AUTOIMMUNITY

Macrophages are certainly key mediators of various immune tolerance mechanisms and are crucial in preventing inflammation and autoimmune diseases. Understandably, alterations in macrophage function should thus promote autoimmune disease progression. In agreement with this postulate, macrophages from autoimmune diabetes-susceptible NOD mice exhibit significant pro-inflammatory phenotype and function when compared to autoimmune diabetes resistant strains [21-23]. Specifically, macrophages from NOD mice show an increase in IL-12 production when co-cultured with T cells, which may lead to an amplification of pathogenic T cells in these mice [23]. Notably, the inflammatory role of macrophages has been revealed in the depletion studies, whereby depletion of macrophages prevents the occurrence of autoimmunity. Indeed, macrophage removal abrogates EAE development in rats and mice [24, 25], as well as endotoxin-induced uveitis [26].

Macrophages also play a central role in the elimination of apoptotic cells. Not surprisingly, there are various experimental evidence that a reduction or modulation of the phagocytosis of apoptotic cells potential of macrophages can result in autoimmunity. For instance, defects in the production of opsonizing molecules such as C1q, MFG-E8 and mannose-binding lectin [7, 10, 27], have been associated with autoimmunity in mice. Modulation of key proteins involved in the apoptotic cell phagocytosis synapse most often results in symptomatic autoimmune phenotypes. Moreover, macrophages in NOD mice show impaired phagocytosis of apoptotic cells. An impairment of apoptotic cell engulfment leads to a reduction of anti-inflammatory cytokines and generate a pro-inflammatory microenvironment. The resulting pro-inflammatory environment can be the product of the secondary necrosis of apoptotic cells. Indeed, an increased number of apoptotic bodies have been found in mice with apoptotic cell clearance defects. Taken together, the experimental evidence highlights the crucial implication of macrophages in the pathogenesis of autoimmune diseases, suggesting a potential contribution of these professional phagocytes in human autoimmune pathologies.

MACROPHAGES AND GENETICS

Genetic studies comparing diabetes-resistant and –susceptible mouse strains have revealed a candidate gene, Nramp1, situated within the *Idd5.2* locus. Nramp, mainly expressed by macrophages, has been identified for its role in resistance to intracellular pathogens, such as *Mycobacterium* or *Salmonella* [28, 29]. It has been demonstrated that Nramp is recruited to the phagosomal membrane following phagocytosis, where it impacts on pathogen replication [30]. Moreover, Nramp1 is necessary for efficient recycling of iron from senescent erythrocytes following phagocytosis by macrophages [31]. Recent work has validated Nramp as an important player in autoimmune disease susceptibility, as autoimmune diabetes incidence was decreased upon *in vivo* silencing Nramp protein expression in mice carrying the *Nramp* autoimmune-susceptibility allele [22]. These results provide an interesting example of where cellular biology meets genetics to validate genes involved in disease susceptibility and progression. Polymorphisms in Nramp, as well as MFG-E8 and C1q, correlate with autoimmune susceptibility in humans, corroborating the murine studies. These data show that the modulation of specific protein function relevant to macrophage biology influence clinical disease predisposition, such as SLE.

CONCLUSION

Macrophages significantly contribute to immune tolerance induction and modulation of their functions may help prevent autoimmune disease progression. Consequently, more work is needed to better understand the biology and genetics of macrophages to establish them as potential therapeutic targets.

REFERENCES

[1] Schulze, C., Munoz, L. E., Franz, S., Sarter, K., Chaurio, R. A., Gaipl, U. S. and Herrmann, M., Clearance deficiency--a potential link between infections and autoimmunity. *Autoimmun. Rev.* 2008. 8: 5-8.

[2] Wermeling, F., Karlsson, M. C. and McGaha, T. L., An anatomical view on macrophages in tolerance. *Autoimmun. Rev.* 2009. 9: 49-52.

[3] Tas, S. W., Quartier, P., Botto, M. and Fossati-Jimack, L., Macrophages from patients with SLE and rheumatoid arthritis have defective adhesion in vitro, while only SLE macrophages have impaired uptake of apoptotic cells. *Ann. Rheum. Dis.* 2006. 65: 216-221.

[4] Lleo, A., Selmi, C., Invernizzi, P., Podda, M. and Gershwin, M. E., The consequences of apoptosis in autoimmunity. *J. Autoimmun.* 2008. 31: 257-262.

[5] Lu, J. H., Teh, B. K., Wang, L., Wang, Y. N., Tan, Y. S., Lai, M. C. and Reid, K. B., The classical and regulatory functions of C1q in immunity and autoimmunity. *Cell Mol. Immunol.* 2008. 5: 9-21.

[6] Gershov, D., Kim, S., Brot, N. and Elkon, K. B., C-Reactive protein binds to apoptotic cells, protects the cells from assembly of the terminal complement components, and sustains an antiinflammatory innate immune response: implications for systemic autoimmunity. *J. Exp. Med.* 2000. 192: 1353-1364.

[7] Botto, M., Dell'Agnola, C., Bygrave, A. E., Thompson, E. M., Cook, H. T., Petry, F., Loos, M., Pandolfi, P. P. and Walport, M. J., Homozygous C1q deficiency causes glomerulonephritis associated with multiple apoptotic bodies. *Nat. Genet.* 1998. 19: 56-59.

[8] Namjou, B., Gray-McGuire, C., Sestak, A. L., Gilkeson, G. S., Jacob, C. O., Merrill, J. T., James, J. A., Wakeland, E. K., Li, Q. Z., Langefeld, C. D., Divers, J., Ziegler, J., Moser, K. L., Kelly, J. A., Kaufman, K. M. and Harley, J. B., Evaluation of C1q genomic region in minority racial groups of lupus. *Genes Immun.* 2009. 10: 517-524.

[9] Martens, H. A., Zuurman, M. W., de Lange, A. H., Nolte, I. M., van der Steege, G., Navis, G. J., Kallenberg, C. G., Seelen, M. A. and Bijl, M., Analysis of C1q polymorphisms suggests association with systemic lupus erythematosus, serum C1q and CH50 levels and disease severity. *Ann. Rheum. Dis.* 2009. 68: 715-720.

[10] Hu, C. Y., Wu, C. S., Tsai, H. F., Chang, S. K., Tsai, W. I. and Hsu, P. N., Genetic polymorphism in milk fat globule-EGF factor 8 (MFG-E8) is associated with systemic lupus erythematosus in human. *Lupus.* 2009. 18: 676-681.

[11] Hanayama, R., Tanaka, M., Miyasaka, K., Aozasa, K., Koike, M., Uchiyama, Y. and Nagata, S., Autoimmune disease and impaired uptake of apoptotic cells in MFG-E8-deficient mice. *Science.* 2004. 304: 1147-1150.

[12] Yamaguchi, H., Takagi, J., Miyamae, T., Yokota, S., Fujimoto, T., Nakamura, S., Ohshima, S., Naka, T. and Nagata, S., Milk fat globule EGF factor 8 in the serum of human patients of systemic lupus erythematosus. *J. Leukoc. Biol.* 2008. 83: 1300-1307.

[13] Matlack, R., Yeh, K., Rosini, L., Gonzalez, D., Taylor, J., Silberman, D., Pennello, A. and Riggs, J., Peritoneal macrophages suppress T-cell activation by amino acid catabolism. *Immunology.* 2006. 117: 386-395.

[14] Gajewski, T. F., Meng, Y. and Harlin, H., Immune suppression in the tumor microenvironment. *J. Immunother.* 2006. 29: 233-240.

[15] Wei, X. Q., Charles, I. G., Smith, A., Ure, J., Feng, G. J., Huang, F. P., Xu, D., Muller, W., Moncada, S. and Liew, F. Y., Altered immune responses in mice lacking inducible nitric oxide synthase. *Nature.* 1995. 375: 408-411.

[16] Kahl, K. G., Schmidt, H. H., Jung, S., Sherman, P., Toyka, K. V. and Zielasek, J., Experimental autoimmune encephalomyelitis in mice with a targeted deletion of the inducible nitric oxide synthase gene: increased T-helper 1 response. *Neurosci. Lett.* 2004. 358: 58-62.

[17] Fenyk-Melody, J. E., Garrison, A. E., Brunnert, S. R., Weidner, J. R., Shen, F., Shelton, B. A. and Mudgett, J. S., Experimental autoimmune encephalomyelitis is exacerbated in mice lacking the NOS2 gene. *J. Immunol.* 1998. 160: 2940-2946.

[18] Hoves, S., Krause, S. W., Schutz, C., Halbritter, D., Scholmerich, J., Herfarth, H. and Fleck, M., Monocyte-derived human macrophages mediate anergy in allogeneic T cells and induce regulatory T cells. *J. Immunol.* 2006. 177: 2691-2698.

[19] Kosiewicz, M. M., Alard, P., Liang, S. and Clark, S. L., Mechanisms of tolerance induced by transforming growth factor-beta-treated antigen-presenting cells: CD8 regulatory T cells inhibit the effector phase of the immune response in primed mice through a mechanism involving Fas ligand. *Int. Immunol.* 2004. 16: 697-706.

[20] Alard, P., Clark, S. L. and Kosiewicz, M. M., Mechanisms of tolerance induced by TGF beta-treated APC: CD4 regulatory T cells prevent the induction of the immune response possibly through a mechanism involving TGF beta. *Eur. J. Immunol.* 2004. 34: 1021-1030.

[21] Shultz, L. D., Schweitzer, P. A., Christianson, S. W., Gott, B., Schweitzer, I. B., Tennent, B., McKenna, S., Mobraaten, L., Rajan, T. V., Greiner, D. L. and et al., Multiple defects in innate and adaptive immunologic function in NOD/LtSz-scid mice. *J. Immunol.* 1995. 154: 180-191.

[22] Kissler, S., Stern, P., Takahashi, K., Hunter, K., Peterson, L. B. and Wicker, L. S., In vivo RNA interference demonstrates a role for Nramp1 in modifying susceptibility to type 1 diabetes. *Nat. Genet.* 2006. 38: 479-483.

[23] Marleau, A. M., Summers, K. L. and Singh, B., Differential Contributions of APC Subsets to T Cell Activation in Nonobese Diabetic Mice. *J. Immunol.* 2008. 180: 5235-5249.

[24] Huitinga, I., van Rooijen, N., de Groot, C. J., Uitdehaag, B. M. and Dijkstra, C. D., Suppression of experimental allergic encephalomyelitis in Lewis rats after elimination of macrophages. *J. Exp. Med.* 1990. 172: 1025-1033.

[25] Tran, E. H., Hoekstra, K., van Rooijen, N., Dijkstra, C. D. and Owens, T., Immune invasion of the central nervous system parenchyma and experimental allergic encephalomyelitis, but not leukocyte extravasation from blood, are prevented in macrophage-depleted mice. *J. Immunol.* 1998. 161: 3767-3775.

[26] Pouvreau, I., Zech, J. C., Thillaye-Goldenberg, B., Naud, M. C., Van Rooijen, N. and de Kozak, Y., Effect of macrophage depletion by liposomes containing dichloromethylene-diphosphonate on endotoxin-induced uveitis. *J. Neuroimmunol.* 1998. 86: 171-181.

[27] Bouwman, L. H., Roep, B. O. and Roos, A., Mannose-binding lectin: clinical implications for infection, transplantation, and autoimmunity. *Hum. Immunol.* 2006. 67: 247-256.

[28] Vidal, S. M., Malo, D., Vogan, K., Skamene, E. and Gros, P., Natural resistance to infection with intracellular parasites: isolation of a candidate for Bcg. *Cell.* 1993. 73: 469-485.

[29] Gruenheid, S., Pinner, E., Desjardins, M. and Gros, P., Natural resistance to infection with intracellular pathogens: the Nramp1 protein is recruited to the membrane of the phagosome. *J. Exp. Med.* 1997. 185: 717-730.

[30] Gruenheid, S. and Gros, P., Genetic susceptibility to intracellular infections: Nramp1, macrophage function and divalent cations transport. *Curr. Opin. Microbiol.* 2000. 3: 43-48.

[31] Soe-Lin, S., Apte, S. S., Andriopoulos, B., Jr., Andrews, M. C., Schranzhofer, M., Kahawita, T., Garcia-Santos, D. and Ponka, P., Nramp1 promotes efficient macrophage recycling of iron following erythrophagocytosis in vivo. *Proc. Natl. Acad. Sci. U. S. A.* 2009. 106: 5960-5965.

Chapter 6

NATURAL KILLER CELLS

Geneviève Chabot-Roy[1], Sylvie Lesage[2] and Fanny Guimont-Desrochers[2]

[1] Maisonneuve-Rosemont Hospital Research Center, Cellular Immunogenetics Unit, Montreal, Quebec, Canada.
[2] University of Montreal, Department of Microbiology and Immunology, Montreal, Quebec, Canada. Maisonneuve-Rosemont Hospital Research Center, Cellular Immunogenetics Unit, Montreal, Quebec, Canada.

INTRODUCTION

Over 30 years ago, large granular lymphocytes were identified and designated "natural killer" (NK) cells in light of their ability to spontaneously eliminate tumour cells and virus-infected cells without prior sensitization [1]. Today, the tumour immunosurveillance capacity of NK cells is a well documented and accepted function of these cells [2]. Indeed, an increase in the incidence of leukemia has been observed in patients exhibiting dysfunctional NK cells, highlighting the importance of NK cells in the prevention of tumours [3]. In this chapter, we will define the unique differentiation pathway of NK cells, elaborate on their ability to discriminate between self-tissue and infected or cancerous cells, address their role in the prevention and promotion of autoimmune disease progression and discuss the genetic associations of the NK cell phenotype and function with autoimmune disease susceptibility.

DIFFERENTIATION OF NK CELLS

NK cells are a minor lymphocyte population (representing 2-10% of total lymphocytes) that do not express the T- or B-cell antigen receptors (hence their early classification as 'null' cells). This ambiguous phenotype posed a number of challenges to the delineation of their differentiation in the bone marrow. It has now been established that NK cells arise from hematopoietic precursors, specifically the early lymphoid progenitors (ELP) and the common lymphoid progenitors (CLP) subsets [4, 5]. Interestingly, NK cells appear to be closely related to T cells, since they can differentiate from the thymic bipotent T/NK cell progenitor [6, 7]. However, they more typically develop in the adult bone marrow, as for B cells. CD122 expression, a component of the IL-15R, is essential for NK cell maturation [8], since IL-15 induces the proliferation and differentiation of NK cells [9], as well as the up-regulation of transcription factors that specify aspects of NK lineage and function, such as Gata-3, IRF-2 and T-bet [10].

It was first believed that NK cells were a homogenous population. However, it was shown that human NK cells can be distinguished into phenotypically and functionally different subsets, based on their levels of expression of CD56 [11] and more recently on the TNF receptor superfamily member, CD27 [12]. In mice, phenotypic characterization has allowed for the identification of at least 4 distinct NK subsets exhibiting different functions, which can be distinguished according to CD27 and CD11b. A $CD11b^{low}CD27^{low}$ phenotype describes the most immature of the mice NK cell subsets [13]. These immature cells subsequently undergo sequential differentiation steps from $CD11b^{low}CD27^{hi}$ to $CD11b^{hi}CD27^{hi}$ and finally to mature and activated $CD11b^{high}CD27^{low}$ NK cells [13]. In agreement with this maturation scenario, the $CD11b^{low}CD27^{hi}$ subset composes the majority of the NK cell population in foetal and neonatal mice [14]. Moreover, $CD11b^{high}$ NK cells express higher levels and a broader variety of NK receptors, such as the Ly49 receptors, they are found enriched in the periphery in adult mice, and they show more potent effector NK cell functions [15].

THE BIOLOGICAL FUNCTION OF NK CELLS

As their name indicates, NK cells are mostly known for their ability to kill target cells. Indeed, upon efficient stimulation, NK cells have the capacity to eliminate tumours and virally-infected cells. They carry out their cytotoxic function through various, non-redundant mechanisms, where their cytotoxic capacity differs depending on the particular NK cell subset and their variegated expression of NK receptors [16]. Indeed, NK cells can spontaneously lyse their targets by releasing perforin and granzyme granules [17, 18], or induce apoptosis of target cells through their expression of death-inducing ligands, such as FASL, TNF, and TRAIL [19-21].

In addition to their killing potential, NK cells can modulate the outcome of adaptive immune responses through cytokine production. Activated NK cells rapidly produce vast amounts of cytokines, including IFN-γ, GM-CSF, and TNF-α, to promote inflammation, and they secrete chemokines, such as MIP-1α, MIP-1β, CCL1, and RANTES [22-24], to recruit lymphocytes and amplify the inflammatory response. Cytokines released by NK cells also promote the maturation of DCs and influence T cell polarization [25]. Therefore, through cytokine production, NK cells create a bridge between innate an adaptive immunity.

NK CELLS AND TARGET CELL RECOGNITION

Mature NK cells play an important role in immunosurveillance. The "missing-self" hypothesis was originally put forth to explain how NK cells recognize target cells lacking MHC class I expression [26]. However, it is now well understood that NK cells recognize their targets by integrating the responses of both inhibitory and activating receptors, which signal respectively through immunoreceptor tyrosine-based inhibitory motifs (ITIM) and activation motifs (ITAM). Generally, inhibitory receptors bind to self-MHC class I molecules, thereby preventing the NK cell response towards healthy self tissue but not towards infected or cancerous cells, where the MHC class I expression is often down-regulated [27]. In addition, ligands for NK cell activating receptors are seldom expressed on healthy tissue, while these ligands are often upregulated on infected and cancer cells. Therefore, by integrating the signalling responses of both inhibitory and activating receptors, NK cells do not lyse healthy tissue but do specifically eliminate tumour and infected cells.

Inhibitory receptors include a family of Ly49 molecules in mice and killer inhibitory receptors (KIR) in humans [28-30]. Both of these families of receptors contain more than 10 members, each of which confers a unique

MHC class I binding specificity [31]. The NK cell population expresses different combinations of inhibitory receptors with different specificity, generating a broad NK cell repertoire to facilitate adequate recognition of the highly polymorphic MHC class I haplotypes *[32, 33]*. For instance, the Ly49 gene cluster is a large family of highly related genes and is also quite polymorphic between various inbred strains of mice. Consequently, NK cells from the 129 as well as the inbred C57BL/6 strains respond differently to intracellular infections, tumour induction, and bone marrow transplantation [34-36]. In addition, the NOD strain has allelic variants of both the 129 and C57BL/6 Ly49 loci, as well as the unique Ly49w gene, which again confers a unique NK cell specificity [37]. These genetic variations have been proposed to contribute to the variability in susceptibility to disease among the different strains [38].

Other than the inhibitory receptors, NK cells express a variety of activating receptors that can modulate their function. By far, NKG2D is the most extensively studied activating receptor. NKG2D ligands, such as MICA/B, ULBPs, Mult1, Rae1, and H60, are normally absent or expressed at a very low level in healthy tissue, but their expression is strongly induced under various pathological conditions [39, 40].

Other NK receptors have also been characterized and include the natural cytotoxicity receptors, NKp30, NKp44, and NKp46 [41-43], the CD94/NKG2A heterodimeric receptor [44], the inhibitory receptor for non-MHC molecules, NKR-P1B [45], and the 2B4 (CD244) activating receptor [46].

In summary, upon maturation, NK cells acquire the expression of several activating and inhibitory receptors, which are dictated both by germline-encoded genetic loci as well as the stromal environment in which the NK cells differentiate [33]. NK cells, thus, compose a heterogeneous population and express a distinct set and level of activating and inhibitory receptors.

NK CELLS IN AUTOIMMUNITY

Because of their capacity to respond promptly, NK cells need to be carefully regulated to prevent damage to healthy tissues, which could lead to autoimmunity. Interestingly, under distinct circumstances, NK cells have been shown to either prevent or promote the development of autoimmune responses.

On the one hand, NK cells have been proposed to play an immunoregulatory protective function, since their numbers and functions are decreased in patients afflicted with MS, SLE, RA, or T1D [47-50]. Moreover, depletion of NK cells in mouse and rat models of MS increases disease severity [51-53]. In one of these studies, it was suggested that NK cells prevent MS development through the elimination of pathogenic CD4+ effector T cells [52]. Moreover, others have demonstrated that NK cells inhibit the proliferation of autoreactive T cells [54]. NK cells have also been proposed to control autoimmunity by killing activated autologous macrophages [55]. The observation that NK cells prevent autoimmune progression has not been limited to models of MS. Indeed, autoimmune diabetes-susceptible NOD mice are protected from disease progression by the administration of complete Freund's adjuvant (CFA), and depletion of NK cells prior to CFA injection abolishes the protective effect [56]. Finally, NK cells also produce Th2 cytokines, such as IL-5, IL-10, and IL-13, which counterbalances the effect of the pro-inflammatory Th1 cytokine, IFNγ, and thus prevents autoimmunity [57-59].

On the other hand, NK cells are cytopathic and induce inflammation and, as such, may contribute to autoimmune disease progression. Evidence in support of their contribution to autoimmunity has been presented in various models. For instance, in a model of myasthenia gravis, NK cell depletion during the priming phase prevents disease onset. In this setting, NK cells are required to mount a Th1 response facilitating the production of pathogenic autoantibodies [60]. NK cells also eliminate pancreatic β cells in a virally-induced model of autoimmune diabetes [61]. Moreover, NK cells have been associated with aggressive insulitis where NK cell depletion reduced the incidence of autoimmune diabetes in NOD mice [62]. In further support of a role for NK cells in autoimmune diabetes progression, NK cells from recently diagnosed diabetic patients showed a high level IFN-γ expression. Interestingly, the NK cell activation state is reduced in long standing patients [63], suggesting that NK cells could participate in the initiation of the disease and become non-functional or exhausted upon chronic stimulation.

Altogether, these reports suggest that NK cells may prevent or promote autoimmunity depending on the disease state, the cytokine milieu, the type of NK cell subset targeted, as well as many other parameters. More work will be needed to decipher the exact contribution of NK cells and NK cell subsets to autoimmune disease progression.

NK Cells and Genetics

Genetic variations in NK cell function and/or receptor expression are associated with autoimmune disease progression. For instance, NK cells from autoimmune-prone NOD mice have poor effector function, supporting the view that adequate NK cell function protects from autoimmune disease progression [64-66]. Moreover, NOD mice overexpress the NKG2D activating ligand, Rae-1, where this phenotype associates with altered NKG2D functions [67]. Similarly, a study on human diabetic patients has also noted a reduced expression of NKG2D as well as a genetic association between a specific MICA allele and disease susceptibility [63]. Together, these results suggest an important role for NKG2D and its ligands in contributing to autoimmune susceptibility.

Genetic susceptibility to autoimmune diseases has been extensively studied using NOD mice and has revealed many genetic loci associated with disease predisposition [68]. In particular, at least one of two genetically linked loci, namely *Idd6* and *Idd19*, is highly relevant to NK cell function. The genetic interval containing these loci is located on chromosome 6 and includes the NK gene complex, which encodes for many NK receptors [69]. Further studies are needed to determine the genetic polymorphism(s) within this interval that directly promote susceptibility to disease. Finally, DAP12, DAP10, and Flt3L, which are important for defining NK cell as well as DC function, are located in the proximal region of chromosome 7, an interval associated with disease susceptibility. Moreover, these genes are differentially expressed between the autoimmune-prone NOD and the autoimmune-resistant C57BL/6 strains [62]. Additional studies are needed to establish their exact role in autoimmune susceptibility.

Conclusion

The contribution of the various facets of NK cells, such as their function, receptor expression, repertoire, subsets, maturation, differentiation, and cytokine production, to autoimmune disease susceptibility remains to be fully elucidated. Until then, this fascinating cell type will continue to intrigue us.

REFERENCES

[1] Kiessling, R., Klein, E., Pross, H. and Wigzell, H., "Natural" killer cells in the mouse. II. Cytotoxic cells with specificity for mouse Moloney leukemia cells. Characteristics of the killer cell. *Eur. J. Immunol.* 1975. 5: 117-121.

[2] Raulet, D. H. and Guerra, N., Oncogenic stress sensed by the immune system: role of natural killer cell receptors. *Nat. Rev. Immunol.* 2009. 9: 568-580.

[3] Smith, B. R., Rosenthal, D. S. and Ault, K. A., Natural killer lymphocytes in hairy cell leukemia: presence of phenotypically identifiable cells with defective functional activity. *Exp. Hematol.* 1985. 13: 189-193.

[4] Igarashi, H., Gregory, S. C., Yokota, T., Sakaguchi, N. and Kincade, P. W., Transcription from the RAG1 locus marks the earliest lymphocyte progenitors in bone marrow. *Immunity.* 2002. 17: 117-130.

[5] Kondo, M., Weissman, I. L. and Akashi, K., Identification of clonogenic common lymphoid progenitors in mouse bone marrow. *Cell.* 1997. 91: 661-672.

[6] Carlyle, J. R., Michie, A. M., Cho, S. K. and Zuniga-Pflucker, J. C., Natural killer cell development and function precede alpha beta T cell differentiation in mouse fetal thymic ontogeny. *J. Immunol.* 1998. 160: 744-753.

[7] Spits, H., Lanier, L. L. and Phillips, J. H., Development of human T and natural killer cells. *Blood.* 1995. 85: 2654-2670.

[8] Di Santo, J. P., Natural killer cell developmental pathways: a question of balance. *Annu. Rev. Immunol.* 2006. 24: 257-286.

[9] Rosmaraki, E. E., Douagi, I., Roth, C., Colucci, F., Cumano, A. and Di Santo, J. P., Identification of committed NK cell progenitors in adult murine bone marrow. *Eur. J. Immunol.* 2001. 31: 1900-1909.

[10] Di Santo, J. P. and Vosshenrich, C. A., Bone marrow versus thymic pathways of natural killer cell development. *Immunol. Rev.* 2006. 214: 35-46.

[11] Sedlmayr, P., Schallhammer, L., Hammer, A., Wilders-Truschnig, M., Wintersteiger, R. and Dohr, G., Differential phenotypic properties of human peripheral blood CD56dim+ and CD56bright+ natural killer cell subpopulations. *Int. Arch. Allergy Immunol.* 1996. 110: 308-313.

[12] Vossen, M. T., Matmati, M., Hertoghs, K. M., Baars, P. A., Gent, M. R., Leclercq, G., Hamann, J., Kuijpers, T. W. and van Lier, R. A., CD27

defines phenotypically and functionally different human NK cell subsets. *J. Immunol.* 2008. 180: 3739-3745.

[13] Chiossone, L., Chaix, J., Fuseri, N., Roth, C., Vivier, E. and Walzer, T., Maturation of mouse NK cells is a 4-stage developmental program. *Blood.* 2009. 113: 5488-5496.

[14] Takeda, K., Cretney, E., Hayakawa, Y., Ota, T., Akiba, H., Ogasawara, K., Yagita, H., Kinoshita, K., Okumura, K. and Smyth, M. J., TRAIL identifies immature natural killer cells in newborn mice and adult mouse liver. *Blood.* 2005. 105: 2082-2089.

[15] Kim, S., Iizuka, K., Kang, H. S., Dokun, A., French, A. R., Greco, S. and Yokoyama, W. M., In vivo developmental stages in murine natural killer cell maturation. *Nat. Immunol.* 2002. 3: 523-528.

[16] Hayakawa, Y., Huntington, N. D., Nutt, S. L. and Smyth, M. J., Functional subsets of mouse natural killer cells. *Immunol. Rev.* 2006. 214: 47-55.

[17] Roder, J. C., Argov, S., Klein, M., Petersson, C., Kiessling, R., Andersson, K. and Hansson, M., Target-effector cell interaction in the natural killer cell system. V. Energy requirements, membrane integrity, and the possible involvement of lysosomal enzymes. *Immunology.* 1980. 40: 107-116.

[18] Dean, J. H., Silva, J. S., Mc, C. J., Leonard, C. M., Cannon, G. B. and Herberman, R. B., Functional activities of rosette separated human peripheral blood leukocytes. *J. Immunol.* 1975. 115: 1449-1455.

[19] Liu, C. C., Walsh, C. M., Eto, N., Clark, W. R. and Young, J. D., Morphologic and functional characterization of perforin-deficient lymphokine-activated killer cells. *J. Immunol.* 1995. 155: 602-608.

[20] Arase, H., Arase, N. and Saito, T., Fas-mediated cytotoxicity by freshly isolated natural killer cells. *J.Exp.Med.*1995. 181: 1235-1238.

[21] Kashii, Y., Giorda, R., Herberman, R. B., Whiteside, T. L. and Vujanovic, N. L., Constitutive expression and role of the TNF family ligands in apoptotic killing of tumor cells by human NK cells. *J. Immunol.* 1999. 163: 5358-5366.

[22] Cooper, M. A., Fehniger, T. A. and Caligiuri, M. A., The biology of human natural killer-cell subsets. *Trends Immunol* 2001. 22: 633-640.

[23] Robertson, M. J., Role of chemokines in the biology of natural killer cells. *J. Leukoc. Biol.* 2002. 71: 173-183.

[24] Cosman, D., Mullberg, J., Sutherland, C. L., Chin, W., Armitage, R., Fanslow, W., Kubin, M. and Chalupny, N. J., ULBPs, novel MHC class

I-related molecules, bind to CMV glycoprotein UL16 and stimulate NK cytotoxicity through the NKG2D receptor. *Immunity.* 2001. 14: 123-133.
[25] Strowig, T., Brilot, F. and Munz, C., Noncytotoxic functions of NK cells: direct pathogen restriction and assistance to adaptive immunity. *J. Immunol.* 2008. 180: 7785-7791.
[26] Karre, K., Ljunggren, H. G., Piontek, G. and Kiessling, R., Selective rejection of H-2-deficient lymphoma variants suggests alternative immune defence strategy. *Nature.* 1986. 319: 675-678.
[27] Garcia-Lora, A., Algarra, I. and Garrido, F., MHC class I antigens, immune surveillance, and tumor immune escape. *J. Cell Physiol.* 2003. 195: 346-355.
[28] Karlhofer, F. M., Ribaudo, R. K. and Yokoyama, W. M., MHC class I alloantigen specificity of Ly-49+ IL-2-activated natural killer cells. *Nature.* 1992. 358: 66-70.
[29] Colonna, M. and Samaridis, J., Cloning of immunoglobulin-superfamily members associated with HLA-C and HLA-B recognition by human natural killer cells. *Science.* 1995. 268: 405-408.
[30] D'Andrea, A., Chang, C., Franz-Bacon, K., McClanahan, T., Phillips, J. H. and Lanier, L. L., Molecular cloning of NKB1. A natural killer cell receptor for HLA-B allotypes. *J. Immunol.* 1995. 155: 2306-2310.
[31] Yokoyama, W. M. and Seaman, W. E., The Ly-49 and NKR-P1 gene families encoding lectin-like receptors on natural killer cells: the NK gene complex. *Annu. Rev. Immunol.* 1993. 11: 613-635.
[32] Brennan, J., Mager, D., Jefferies, W. and Takei, F., Expression of different members of the Ly-49 gene family defines distinct natural killer cell subsets and cell adhesion properties. *J. Exp. Med.* 1994. 180: 2287-2295.
[33] Raulet, D. H., Held, W., Correa, I., Dorfman, J. R., Wu, M. F. and Corral, L., Specificity, tolerance and developmental regulation of natural killer cells defined by expression of class I-specific Ly49 receptors. *Immunol. Rev.* 1997. 155: 41-52.
[34] Mo, X. Y., Sangster, M., Sarawar, S., Coleclough, C. and Doherty, P. C., Differential antigen burden modulates the gamma interferon but not the immunoglobulin response in mice that vary in susceptibility to Sendai virus pneumonia. *J. Virol.* 1995. 69: 5592-5598.
[35] Mayer, A., Lilly, F. and Duran-Reynals, M. L., Genetically dominant resistance in mice to 3-methylcholanthrene-induced lymphoma. *Proc. Natl. Acad. Sci. U. S. A.* 1980. 77: 2960-2963.

[36] Lotzova, E., Dicke, K. A., Trentin, J. J. and Gallagher, M. T., Genetic control of bone marrow transplantation in irradiated mice: classification of mouse strains according to their responsiveness to bone marrow allografts and xenografts. *Transplant. Proc.* 1977. 9: 289-292.

[37] Silver, E. T., Gong, D., Hazes, B. and Kane, K. P., Ly-49W, an activating receptor of nonobese diabetic mice with close homology to the inhibitory receptor Ly-49G, recognizes H-2D(k) and H-2D(d). *J. Immunol.* 2001. 166: 2333-2341.

[38] Makrigiannis, A. P. and Anderson, S. K., Regulation of natural killer cell function. *Cancer Biol. Ther.* 2003. 2: 610-616.

[39] Groh, V., Rhinehart, R., Secrist, H., Bauer, S., Grabstein, K. H. and Spies, T., Broad tumor-associated expression and recognition by tumor-derived gamma delta T cells of MICA and MICB. *Proc. Natl. Acad. Sci. U. S. A.* 1999. 96: 6879-6884.

[40] Diefenbach, A., Jensen, E. R., Jamieson, A. M. and Raulet, D. H., Rae1 and H60 ligands of the NKG2D receptor stimulate tumour immunity. *Nature.* 2001. 413: 165-171.

[41] Pende, D., Parolini, S., Pessino, A., Sivori, S., Augugliaro, R., Morelli, L., Marcenaro, E., Accame, L., Malaspina, A., Biassoni, R., Bottino, C., Moretta, L. and Moretta, A., Identification and molecular characterization of NKp30, a novel triggering receptor involved in natural cytotoxicity mediated by human natural killer cells. *J. Exp. Med.* 1999. 190: 1505-1516.

[42] Vitale, M., Bottino, C., Sivori, S., Sanseverino, L., Castriconi, R., Marcenaro, E., Augugliaro, R., Moretta, L. and Moretta, A., NKp44, a novel triggering surface molecule specifically expressed by activated natural killer cells, is involved in non-major histocompatibility complex-restricted tumor cell lysis. *J. Exp. Med.* 1998. 187: 2065-2072.

[43] Sivori, S., Vitale, M., Morelli, L., Sanseverino, L., Augugliaro, R., Bottino, C., Moretta, L. and Moretta, A., p46, a novel natural killer cell-specific surface molecule that mediates cell activation. *J. Exp. Med.* 1997. 186: 1129-1136.

[44] Moretta, A., Vitale, M., Sivori, S., Bottino, C., Morelli, L., Augugliaro, R., Barbaresi, M., Pende, D., Ciccone, E., Lopez-Botet, M. and Moretta, L., Human natural killer cell receptors for HLA-class I molecules. Evidence that the Kp43 (CD94) molecule functions as receptor for HLA-B alleles. *J. Exp. Med.* 1994. 180: 545-555.

[45] Carlyle, J. R., Martin, A., Mehra, A., Attisano, L., Tsui, F. W. and Zuniga-Pflucker, J. C., Mouse NKR-P1B, a novel NK1.1 antigen with inhibitory function. *J. Immunol.* 1999. 162: 5917-5923.
[46] Brown, M. H., Boles, K., van der Merwe, P. A., Kumar, V., Mathew, P. A. and Barclay, A. N., 2B4, the natural killer and T cell immunoglobulin superfamily surface protein, is a ligand for CD48. *J. Exp. Med.* 1998. 188: 2083-2090.
[47] Grunebaum, E., Malatzky-Goshen, E. and Shoenfeld, Y., Natural killer cells and autoimmunity. *Immunol. Res.* 1989. 8: 292-304.
[48] Baxter, A. G. and Smyth, M. J., The role of NK cells in autoimmune disease. *Autoimmunity.* 2002. 35: 1-14.
[49] Shibatomi, K., Ida, H., Yamasaki, S., Nakashima, T., Origuchi, T., Kawakami, A., Migita, K., Kawabe, Y., Tsujihata, M., Anderson, P. and Eguchi, K., A novel role for interleukin-18 in human natural killer cell death: high serum levels and low natural killer cell numbers in patients with systemic autoimmune diseases. *Arthritis Rheum.* 2001. 44: 884-892.
[50] Grom, A. A., Villanueva, J., Lee, S., Goldmuntz, E. A., Passo, M. H. and Filipovich, A., Natural killer cell dysfunction in patients with systemic-onset juvenile rheumatoid arthritis and macrophage activation syndrome. *J. Pediatr.* 2003. 142: 292-296.
[51] Hammarberg, H., Lidman, O., Lundberg, C., Eltayeb, S. Y., Gielen, A. W., Muhallab, S., Svenningsson, A., Linda, H., van Der Meide, P. H., Cullheim, S., Olsson, T. and Piehl, F., Neuroprotection by encephalomyelitis: rescue of mechanically injured neurons and neurotrophin production by CNS-infiltrating T and natural killer cells. *J. Neurosci.* 2000. 20: 5283-5291.
[52] Zhang, B., Yamamura, T., Kondo, T., Fujiwara, M. and Tabira, T., Regulation of experimental autoimmune encephalomyelitis by natural killer (NK) cells. *J. Exp. Med.* 1997. 186: 1677-1687.
[53] Matsumoto, Y., Kohyama, K., Aikawa, Y., Shin, T., Kawazoe, Y., Suzuki, Y. and Tanuma, N., Role of natural killer cells and TCR gamma delta T cells in acute autoimmune encephalomyelitis. *Eur. J. Immunol.* 1998. 28: 1681-1688.
[54] Smeltz, R. B., Wolf, N. A. and Swanborg, R. H., Inhibition of autoimmune T cell responses in the DA rat by bone marrow-derived NK cells in vitro: implications for autoimmunity. *J. Immunol.* 1999. 163: 1390-1397.

[55] Nedvetzki, S., Sowinski, S., Eagle, R. A., Harris, J., Vely, F., Pende, D., Trowsdale, J., Vivier, E., Gordon, S. and Davis, D. M., Reciprocal regulation of human natural killer cells and macrophages associated with distinct immune synapses. *Blood.* 2007. 109: 3776-3785.

[56] Lee, I. F., Qin, H., Trudeau, J., Dutz, J. and Tan, R., Regulation of autoimmune diabetes by complete Freund's adjuvant is mediated by NK cells. *J. Immunol.* 2004. 172: 937-942.

[57] Colucci, F., Di Santo, J. P. and Leibson, P. J., Natural killer cell activation in mice and men: different triggers for similar weapons? *Nat. Immunol.* 2002. 3: 807-813.

[58] Loza, M. J., Zamai, L., Azzoni, L., Rosati, E. and Perussia, B., Expression of type 1 (interferon gamma) and type 2 (interleukin-13, interleukin-5) cytokines at distinct stages of natural killer cell differentiation from progenitor cells. *Blood.* 2002. 99: 1273-1281.

[59] Lauwerys, B. R., Garot, N., Renauld, J. C. and Houssiau, F. A., Cytokine production and killer activity of NK/T-NK cells derived with IL-2, IL-15, or the combination of IL-12 and IL-18. *J. Immunol.* 2000. 165: 1847-1853.

[60] Shi, F. D., Wang, H. B., Li, H., Hong, S., Taniguchi, M., Link, H., Van Kaer, L. and Ljunggren, H. G., Natural killer cells determine the outcome of B cell-mediated autoimmunity. *Nat. Immunol.* 2000. 1: 245-251.

[61] Flodstrom, M., Maday, A., Balakrishna, D., Cleary, M. M., Yoshimura, A. and Sarvetnick, N., Target cell defense prevents the development of diabetes after viral infection. *Nat. Immunol.* 2002. 3: 373-382.

[62] Poirot, L., Benoist, C. and Mathis, D., Natural killer cells distinguish innocuous and destructive forms of pancreatic islet autoimmunity. *Proc. Natl. Acad. Sci. U. S. A.* 2004. 101: 8102-8107.

[63] Rodacki, M., Svoren, B., Butty, V., Besse, W., Laffel, L., Benoist, C. and Mathis, D., Altered natural killer cells in type 1 diabetic patients. *Diabetes.* 2007. 56: 177-185.

[64] Carnaud, C., Gombert, J., Donnars, O., Garchon, H. and Herbelin, A., Protection against diabetes and improved NK/NKT cell performance in NOD.NK1.1 mice congenic at the NK complex. *J. Immunol.* 2001. 166: 2404-2411.

[65] Poulton, L. D., Smyth, M. J., Hawke, C. G., Silveira, P., Shepherd, D., Naidenko, O. V., Godfrey, D. I. and Baxter, A. G., Cytometric and functional analyses of NK and NKT cell deficiencies in NOD mice. *Int. Immunol.* 2001. 13: 887-896.

[66] Johansson, S. E., Hall, H., Bjorklund, J. and Hoglund, P., Broadly impaired NK cell function in non-obese diabetic mice is partially restored by NK cell activation in vivo and by IL-12/IL-18 in vitro. *Int. Immunol.* 2004. 16: 1-11.

[67] Ogasawara, K., Hamerman, J. A., Hsin, H., Chikuma, S., Bour-Jordan, H., Chen, T., Pertel, T., Carnaud, C., Bluestone, J. A. and Lanier, L. L., Impairment of NK cell function by NKG2D modulation in NOD mice. *Immunity.* 2003. 18: 41-51.

[68] Wicker, L. S., Todd, J. A. and Peterson, L. B., Genetic control of autoimmune diabetes in the NOD mouse. *Annu. Rev. Immunol.* 1995. 13: 179-200.

[69] Rogner, U. C., Boitard, C., Morin, J., Melanitou, E. and Avner, P., Three loci on mouse chromosome 6 influence onset and final incidence of type I diabetes in NOD.C3H congenic strains. *Genomics.* 2001. 74: 163-171.

CLOSING REMARKS

Autoimmune susceptibility is multigenic and is determined by the sum of genetic variants found within an individual. Several possibilities may explain the evolution of such genetic variants. One assumption is that these variants arose from inappropriate genetic recombinations. An alternative scenario is that they were selected over time by natural selection processes to enhance the individual's protection against specific pathogens. Genetic variants may, therefore, increase the reactivity of the immune system and it is the accumulation of these genetic variants within a given person which increases their risk of developing an autoimmune syndrome. As a result, the immune system must find a balance between tolerance to self and reactivity to non-self. This balance is interdependent on the environment, such as pathogens, where stronger immune responses promote survival of the individual but may also lead to autoimmune diseases, whereas weaker immune responses may result in inefficient elimination of pathogens, which can be fatal.

Finally, we are entering an interesting era where genetics meets biology and biology meets genetics in the attempt to decipher the susceptibility to complex disease traits. Collaboration between geneticists and immunobiologists should help unravel the mysteries behind susceptibility to autoimmune diseases. The specific contribution of given cellular pathways to disease susceptibility will most certainly reveal new drug targets in the modulation of responses. An integration of the whole system's biology approaches and genetic information will most certainly prove useful. It should be noted, however, that in developed countries the incidence of autoimmune diseases is rising faster than can be simply explained by the natural selection of genetic variants. This suggests that environmental factors are most probably at play. Therefore, not only should we focus on defining the contribution of each genetic factor associated with disease susceptibility, but it will also be imperative to examine their interaction with environment.

In closing, I would like to thank all my collaborators to this project, including Dr. Adrian Liston and Dr. James R. Carlyle for their respective contributions to chapters 1 and 6.

Sylvie Lesage

INDEX

A

accelerator, x, 31
access, 7
accessibility, 2
acid, 21, 49, 52
acquired immunity, 33
activation state, 59
adhesion, 51, 63
adhesion properties, 63
adulthood, 2
age, 14, 16, 31
allele, 3, 50, 60
alters, 15
antibody, 19, 32
antigen, ix, 12, 13, 15, 20, 21, 22, 27, 28, 29, 31, 32, 35, 37, 39, 40, 44, 45, 53, 56, 63, 65
antigen-presenting cell, 12, 20, 45, 53
APC, ix, 12, 14, 15, 21, 32, 37, 41, 53
apoptosis, 11, 13, 16, 19, 28, 40, 43, 51, 57
arrest, 16
arthritis, 29, 33, 34
autoantibodies, 13, 29, 30, 48, 59
autoantigens, 29
autoimmune disease, vii, 1, 3, 4, 7, 12, 13, 14, 15, 16, 18, 19, 20, 22, 23, 28, 29, 30, 32, 33, 35, 38, 40, 41, 49, 50, 51, 55, 59, 60, 65, 69
autoimmunity, 4, 8, 9, 16, 17, 18, 19, 20, 21, 23, 24, 29, 30, 32, 33, 34, 35, 37, 38, 41, 43, 48, 50, 51, 52, 54, 58, 59, 65, 66
autosomal recessive, 13
availability, 3, 5, 28

B

Baars, 61
background, 13
bacterial infection, 43
binding, 12, 16, 23, 48, 50, 54, 58
biological processes, 1
biological systems, 2
blood, 54
bone, 28, 56, 58, 61, 64, 65
bone marrow, 28, 56, 58, 61, 64, 65
bone marrow transplant, 58, 64
brain, 13, 24
breakdown, 4, 30

C

Canada, 1, 11, 27, 37, 47, 55
cancer, 37, 57
cancer cells, 57
cancerous cells, 55, 57
cardiomyopathy, 16
catabolism, 49, 52
CD8+, 44

cell, vii, ix, 1, 2, 11, 12, 14, 15, 18, 23, 24, 27, 28, 29, 30, 31, 32, 33, 34, 35, 37, 38, 39, 40, 41, 42, 43, 45, 48, 49, 50, 52, 55, 56, 57, 58, 59, 60, 61, 62, 63, 64, 65, 66, 67
cell cycle, 16
cell death, ix, 13, 16, 43
cell killing, 48
cell line, 2
cell lines, 2
central nervous system, 53
challenges, 9, 56
chemokines, 57, 62
chromosome, 4, 5, 31, 40, 60, 67
circulation, 16
classification, 56, 64
clinical symptoms, 2
cloning, 63
CNS, 24, 65
coding, 3
colitis, x
complement, 48, 51
components, 3, 51
Congress, iv
control, 11, 14, 16, 20, 22, 25, 31, 44, 59, 64, 67
conversion, 48
Copyright, iv
CSF, 57
cytokines, 14, 17, 18, 24, 28, 29, 30, 34, 48, 50, 57, 59, 66
cytotoxicity, 58, 62, 63, 64

D

damages, iv
danger, 47, 48
death, x, 16, 57, 65
defects, vii, 11, 13, 15, 16, 30, 38, 43, 50, 53
defence, 63
defense, 66
deficiencies, 2, 13, 20, 39, 66
deficiency, 16, 19, 22, 43, 51, 52

dendritic cell, vii, ix, x, 12, 32, 33, 38, 40, 41, 42, 43, 44, 45, 46, 48
deprivation, 14
destruction, 22
developed countries, 69
deviation, 17
diabetes, vii, ix, x, 4, 6, 9, 11, 13, 15, 16, 17, 18, 19, 21, 22, 24, 25, 31, 35, 39, 40, 41, 43, 44, 46, 49, 50, 59, 66, 67
diabetic patients, 59, 60, 66
dichotomy, 18
differentiation, 14, 17, 21, 24, 29, 33, 38, 39, 42, 49, 55, 56, 60, 61, 66
dilated cardiomyopathy, 23
discrimination, 12
disease progression, 15, 18, 30, 32, 49, 59, 60
diseases, vii, 1, 3, 4, 5, 7, 8, 9, 10, 11, 16, 18, 28, 69
disequilibrium, x, 3, 5
distribution, 41, 42
diversity, 24, 45
DNA, 3, 5, 33
dosage, 20
Drosophila, 2, 8
drug targets, 69
duplication, 35

E

EAE, ix, 24, 29, 49, 50
embryology, 2
encephalomyelitis, 52, 53, 65
encoding, 23, 63
endocrine, 2
engagement, 24, 33
environment, 50, 58, 69, 70
environmental factors, 6, 69
enzymes, 49, 62
epithelial cells, x, 12, 19
erythrocytes, 50
ethnic groups, 6
evolution, 69
execution, 2

experimental autoimmune
  encephalomyelitis, ix, 29, 65
extravasation, 53

F

false positive, 6
family, 13, 19, 22, 24, 28, 31, 44, 57, 62, 63
fat, 48, 52
feedback, 24
Ford, 21
France, 11

G

gene, 2, 3, 4, 5, 6, 14, 16, 17, 19, 20, 23, 24, 31, 34, 35, 50, 53, 58, 60, 63
gene expression, 2, 4, 24
generation, 7, 14, 17, 40, 44, 45, 49
genes, 1, 2, 3, 4, 5, 6, 7, 8, 30, 32, 34, 40, 51, 58, 60
genetic defect, 14
genetic factors, 1, 2, 7
genetic information, 69
genetic traits, 1, 4
genetics, 2, 3, 5, 7, 8, 9, 51, 69
genome, vii, ix, 2, 3, 5, 8, 9, 18
genotype, 3, 5, 7, 9
glomerulonephritis, 48, 52
glycosylation, 21
granules, 57
groups, 3, 15, 52

H

hairy cell leukemia, 61
haplotypes, 5, 58
heritability, 10
heterogeneity, 3
histology, 24
HLA, ix, 4, 5, 9, 63, 64
homeostasis, 22
host, 12
human condition, 2
human genome, 2, 4, 6
humoral immunity, 33
Hunter, 8, 10, 20, 22, 23, 45, 53
hyperactivity, 31
hypothesis, 23, 31, 57

I

ICD, 16
identification, vii, 1, 3, 6, 7, 13, 40, 56
IFN, ix, 17, 24, 28, 33, 40, 44, 45, 46, 57, 59
IL-13, 59
IL-17, 11, 17, 24
IL-6, 17, 24
IL-8, 17
immune activation, 38
immune function, 37
immune regulation, 14, 18, 34
immune response, 1, 12, 15, 17, 18, 27, 37, 47, 52, 53, 57, 69
immune system, vii, 1, 2, 27, 32, 37, 48, 61, 69
immunity, 37, 45, 51, 57, 63, 64
immunoglobulin, 27, 32, 63, 65
immunoglobulin superfamily, 65
immunosurveillance, 55, 57
immunotherapy, 35
in vitro, 42, 51, 65, 67
in vivo, 22, 32, 33, 39, 42, 43, 44, 45, 49, 50, 54, 67
incidence, 50, 55, 59, 67, 69
indicators, 3
indirect effect, 28
induction, 12, 13, 15, 17, 18, 19, 20, 22, 24, 31, 38, 39, 40, 41, 42, 48, 49, 51, 53, 58
infection, 47, 54
inflammation, 1, 13, 15, 24, 29, 39, 44, 47, 48, 49, 57, 59
inflammatory responses, 17, 39
inhibition, 16, 18, 24
inhibitor, 16
initiation, 59
injury, iv
INS, 4

insulin, 4, 15
integration, 69
integrin, 39
integrity, 62
interaction, 13, 15, 47, 62, 70
interference, 23, 53
interferon (IFN), ix, 28, 33, 40, 44, 45, 63, 66
interferon gamma, 66
interferons, 33
interleukin-17, 18
interval, 17, 40, 60
iron, 50, 54
isolation, 54

J

Jordan, 67
juvenile rheumatoid arthritis, 65

K

kidney, 13
killer cells, 61, 62, 65, 66
killing, 1, 57, 59, 62

L

leukemia, 55, 61
ligand, 15, 23, 38, 43, 53, 60, 65
likelihood, 7
limitation, vii, 5, 6
linkage, x, 3, 4, 5, 6, 9, 40
liposomes, 54
liver, 62
locus, vii, 4, 15, 16, 21, 22, 25, 31, 50, 61
low risk, 1, 4
lupus, 5, 16, 23, 30, 31, 34, 35, 52
lymph, 21, 39
lymph node, 22, 39
lymphocytes, 4, 14, 15, 27, 32, 35, 47, 55, 56, 57, 61
lymphoid, ix, 12, 15, 39, 41, 42, 43, 44, 56, 61
lymphoid organs, 12, 15, 41, 42, 43
lymphoma, 63
lysis, 64

M

macrophages, vii, 12, 17, 29, 41, 47, 48, 49, 50, 51, 52, 53, 59, 66
maintenance, 14, 16, 30, 42, 43, 48
major histocompatibility complex, 44, 64
majority, 5, 18, 56
marrow, 56, 61, 64
maturation, 14, 18, 27, 28, 45, 56, 57, 58, 60, 62
measures, 5
membership, 9
memory, 17, 27, 33, 34
men, 66
metabolites, 49
methodology, 5
MHC, x, 4, 9, 12, 14, 15, 18, 32, 34, 39, 40, 57, 58, 62, 63
mice, 3, 4, 6, 13, 14, 16, 17, 19, 21, 22, 23, 24, 25, 31, 32, 34, 35, 38, 39, 40, 41, 42, 43, 44, 46, 48, 49, 50, 52, 53, 54, 56, 57, 59, 60, 62, 63, 64, 66, 67
milk, 48, 52
minority, 52
MIP, 57
model, 2, 13, 14, 15, 19, 29, 34, 43, 59
models, 2, 6, 40, 59
molecules, 12, 15, 17, 18, 29, 39, 40, 42, 48, 50, 57, 58, 63, 64
motif, 23
multiple sclerosis, 1, 9, 34
mutagen, 3
mutagenesis, 8
mutant, 2
mutation, 14
myasthenia gravis, 59

N

natural killer cell, 61, 62, 63, 64, 65, 66

natural selection, 69
natural selection processes, 69
necrosis, x, 28, 50
neglect, 29
neurons, 2, 65
neutrophils, 17
New Zealand, 34
nitric oxide, ix, 49, 52, 53
nitric oxide synthase, ix, 49, 52, 53
NK cells, vii, 55, 56, 57, 58, 59, 60, 62, 63, 65, 66

O

oligodendrocytes, 1
opportunities, 20
order, 2, 3, 4, 5, 7, 15, 16, 18, 29, 32, 40, 48
organ, 8, 12, 14, 16, 20
organism, 1
oxidative stress, 46

P

pairing, 32
pancreas, 13
parallel, 6
parameters, 59
parenchyma, 53
parity, 21
pathogenesis, 5, 39, 50
pathogens, 12, 47, 48, 50, 54, 69
pathology, 13
pathways, vii, 5, 6, 7, 15, 16, 17, 18, 23, 24, 61, 69
pattern recognition, x, 29
penetrance, 6
peptides, 4, 12
performance, 66
peripheral blood, 61, 62
permission, iv
phagocytosis, 48, 50
phenotype, 2, 7, 14, 24, 38, 40, 48, 49, 55, 56, 60
plasma, 27, 29, 33

plasma cells, 29
plasticity, 33
pneumonia, 63
point mutation, 3
polarization, 57
polymorphism, x, 52, 60
polymorphisms, 3, 5, 17, 21, 48, 49, 52
poor, 60
population, 3, 5, 6, 14, 35, 39, 47, 56, 58
power, 8
prevention, 7, 12, 15, 16, 41, 55
priming, 43, 45, 59
probability, 4
production, 16, 17, 30, 31, 32, 48, 49, 50, 57, 59, 60, 65, 66
program, 14, 62
pro-inflammatory, 17, 29, 48, 49, 50, 59
project, 70
proliferation, 14, 28, 29, 49, 56, 59
properties, 42, 61
proteins, 12, 16, 18, 48, 50

R

range, 1, 3
RANTES, 57
reactions, 12
reactivity, 69
receptors, x, 29, 32, 33, 47, 56, 57, 58, 60, 61, 63, 64
recognition, 1, 12, 15, 18, 58, 63, 64
recombination, 5, 7
recommendations, iv
recycling, 50, 54
regeneration, 46
region, 3, 5, 6, 9, 15, 23, 31, 35, 52, 60
regulation, 14, 16, 17, 18, 19, 29, 30, 31, 33, 56, 63, 66
regulators, 14
rejection, 63
relevance, 2
remission, 49
replication, 6, 50
reproduction, 6
resistance, 19, 21, 40, 43, 50, 54, 63

responsiveness, 28, 64
rewards, 9
rheumatoid arthritis, x, 4, 51
rights, iv
risk, 3, 4, 6, 14, 18, 23, 69
rituximab, 32
RNA, 23, 31, 35, 53

S

sampling, 6
sclerosis, x
scores, 5
search, 12
secrete, 17, 28, 40, 57
secretion, 14, 29, 48
sensitivity, 4, 31
sensitization, 55
serum, 52, 65
severity, 16, 31, 52, 59
shares, 40
signaling pathway, 28
signalling, x, 30, 31, 57
signals, 15, 23, 31, 33
skin, 13
SNP, x, 3
spleen, 37, 39, 42
stabilization, 24
strain, 13, 17, 58
strategies, 2
strategy, vii, 2, 3, 39, 63
strength, 13
stress, 61
stroma, 22
stromal cells, 15
Sun, 21
suppression, 28, 49, 52
surveillance, 63
survival, 12, 18, 28, 38, 69
susceptibility, vii, 1, 2, 3, 4, 5, 6, 7, 8, 9, 10, 11, 13, 15, 16, 17, 18, 23, 30, 31, 34, 35, 40, 49, 50, 53, 54, 55, 58, 60, 63, 69
switching, 33
synapse, 50
syndrome, 20, 30, 65, 69

systemic lupus erythematosus, x, 1, 9, 34, 35, 52

T

T cell, x, 11, 12, 13, 14, 15, 16, 17, 18, 19, 20, 21, 22, 23, 24, 25, 29, 30, 31, 33, 34, 37, 38, 39, 40, 43, 44, 48, 49, 50, 53, 56, 57, 59, 61, 64, 65
T lymphocytes, 11, 12, 15, 49
targets, 57
TCR, x, 13, 15, 21, 38, 65
testing, 5
TGF, 14, 20, 48, 49, 53
therapeutic approaches, 5, 31, 37, 38
therapeutic targets, vii, 17, 51
therapy, 35
threshold, 6, 13, 16
thresholds, 13
thymus, 12, 13, 14, 15, 18, 19, 42
thyroiditis, 11, 13, 19, 30
tissue, x, 1, 2, 13, 16, 22, 23, 41, 44, 47, 48, 55, 57, 58
TLR, 29, 30, 33, 34
TLR9, 33
TNF, x, 17, 28, 56, 57, 62
traits, 2, 3, 8, 40, 69
transcription, 14, 20, 39, 56
transcription factors, 39, 56
transforming growth factor, 53
translation, vii
translocation, 31, 35
transplantation, 54
transport, 39, 54
treatment methods, 41
triggers, 43, 66
tryptophan, 49
tumor, 1, 46, 52, 62, 63, 64
tumor cells, 1, 46, 62
tumours, 40, 55, 57
turnover, 48
type 1 diabetes, 1, 9, 10, 15, 21, 23, 25, 53
tyrosine, ix, 43, 57

U

ulcerative colitis, 4
uveitis, 50, 54

V

validation, 4
variability, 58
variations, vii, 3, 7, 58, 60
viral infection, 25, 40, 66
virus infection, 33

W

weapons, 66

X

xenografts, 64

Y

Y chromosome, x, 31

Z

zinc, 19